**Pain and Depression**

# Advances in Psychosomatic Medicine

## Vol. 25

Series Editor

*T.N. Wise*  *Falls Church, Va.*

Editors

*G.A. Fava*  *Bologna*
*I. Fukunishi*  *Tokyo*
*M.B. Rosenthal*  *Cleveland, Ohio*

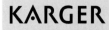

# Pain and Depression

**An Interdisciplinary Patient-Centered Approach**

Volume Editors

*M.R. Clark*   Baltimore, Md.
*G.J. Treisman*   Baltimore, Md.

11 figures and 17 tables, 2004

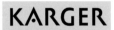

KARGER

Basel · Freiburg · Paris · London · New York ·
Bangalore · Bangkok · Singapore · Tokyo · Sydney

# Advances in Psychosomatic Medicine

Founded 1960 by
F. Deutsch (Cambridge, Mass.)
A. Jores (Hamburg)
B. Stockvis (Leiden)

Continued 1972–1982 by
F. Reichsman (Brooklyn, N.Y.)

Library of Congress Cataloging-in-Publication Data

A catalog record for this title is available from the Library of Congress.

Bibliographic Indices. This publication is listed in bibliographic services, including Current Contents® and Index Medicus.

© Copyright 2004 by S. Karger AG, P.O. Box, CH–4009 Basel (Switzerland)
www.karger.com
Printed in Switzerland on acid-free paper by Reinhardt Druck, Basel
ISSN 0065–3268
ISBN 3–8055–7742–7

# Contents

**VII** Preface

  **1** Perspectives on Pain and Depression
Clark, M.R.; Treisman, G.J. (Baltimore, Md.)

 **28** The Psychological Behaviorism Theory of Pain and the Placebo:
Its Principles and Results of Research Application
Staats, P.S. (Baltimore, Md.); Hekmat, H. (Stevens Point, Wisc.);
Staats, A.W. (Manoa, Hawaii)

 **41** Function, Disability, and Psychological Well-Being
Katz, P. (San Francisco, Calif.)

 **63** Structural Models of Comorbidity among Common
Mental Disorders: Connections to Chronic Pain
Krueger, R.F.; Tackett, J.L.; Markon, K.E. (Minneapolis, Minn.)

 **78** Neurobiology of Pain
Clark, M.R.; Treisman, G.J. (Baltimore, Md.)

 **89** Complex Regional Pain Syndrome: Diagnostic Controversies,
Psychological Dysfunction, and Emerging Concepts
Grabow, T.S.; Christo, P.J.; Raja, S.N. (Baltimore, Md.)

**102 Can We Prevent a Second 'Gulf War Syndrome'? Population-Based Healthcare for Chronic Idiopathic Pain and Fatigue after War**
Engel, C.C. (Bethesda, Md./Washington, D.C.); Jaffer, A.; Adkins, J. (Washington, D.C.); Riddle, J.R.; Gibson R. (Falls Church, Va.)

**123 Opioid Effectiveness, Addiction, and Depression in Chronic Pain**
Christo, P.J.; Grabow, T.S.; Raja, S.N. (Baltimore, Md.)

**138 Opioid Prescribing for Chronic Nonmalignant Pain in Primary Care: Challenges and Solutions**
Olsen, Y.; Daumit, G.L. (Baltimore, Md.)

**151 To Help and Not to Harm: Ethical Issues in the Treatment of Chronic Pain in Patients with Substance Use Disorders**
Geppert, C.M.A. (Albuquerque, N.Mex.)

**172 Subject Index**

......................

# Preface

Pain has become an important topic in medical care as the media have highlighted doctors undertreating pain in dying cancer patients, while at the same time reporting that OxyContin® has become the most abused drug in the United States. Much of the confusion about treatment of pain comes from inadequate evaluation and understanding of pain and a lack of knowledge about the psychiatric conditions that accompany many pain disorders. The distinction between chronic and acute pain syndromes, as well as the distinction between those in whom the goal of treatment is rehabilitation and those who need to be made comfortable has been poorly appreciated in clinical efforts. The idea that pain must be assessed daily in all patients at every clinical interaction and treated with an opiate-based protocol has caused as many problems as it has solved. Acute pain with a known etiology that is expected in the course of treatment should be vigorously suppressed in most cases. Acute pain of unclear etiology should be evaluated for cause and appropriate treatment. Chronic pain in a dying cancer patient should be vigorously suppressed. Chronic pain in most patients deserves a comprehensive workup and thoughtful treatment plan which balances comfort with function and rehabilitation.

Depression is the second most debilitating chronic medical condition. It occurs at high rates in many chronic medical conditions and has been shown to affect recovery, cost, morbidity, and mortality. Depression is often missed in medical settings and is underdiagnosed and undertreated in most studied patient populations. It adds to the costs of treatment, magnifies the subjective experience of noxious stimuli, and retards rehabilitation. Depression is a barrier to patients' engagement in treatment, and sometimes a barrier to physician engagement in patient care. The co-occurrence of these two conditions is well known but the details of phenomenology, interrelationships, and rational therapies remain speculative. This volume focuses on the need for a coherent approach to the formulation of patients with chronic pain who suffer from depression. Depression, just like pain, means many things to many people. Depression is a personal experience that takes on many forms and emerges from many causes.

The Pain Treatment Programs in the Department of Psychiatry and Behavioral Sciences at the Johns Hopkins Medical Institutions have implemented a comprehensive approach to the treatment of patients with chronic pain based on the formulation of each patient's problems. This formulation recognizes that distress and suffering need to be both explained and understood from several different perspectives. These perspectives organize what we know about patients, both from experience and research, into the different kinds of altered circumstances that affect individuals. Each perspective offers a distinct but complementary way in which mental life can become disordered. Clark and Treisman discuss these perspectives and their application to patients with chronic pain in the first paper, 'Perspectives on Pain and Depression'. This discussion is complemented by Staats et al. who present an interdisciplinary structure in their paper, 'The Psychological Behaviorism Theory of Pain and the Placebo: Its Principles and Results of Research Application'.

The recognition that depression is not just an affective disorder or demoralization is discussed in detail in the papers by Katz, 'Function, Disability, and Psychological Well-Being' and Krueger et al., 'Structural Models of Comorbidity among Common Mental Disorders: Connections to Chronic Pain'. Katz explores the relationship between function and well-being recognizing that disability in valued life activities produces depressive symptoms. Specifically, this model addresses the individual's unique interests and wants that chronic pain compromises. Krueger et al. resist the traditional conception of depression as a categorical entity presenting evidence that depression can be explained by dimensional traits that predispose individuals to specific forms of psychopathology. The inherent traits of internalizing and externalizing ultimately generate a variety of psychiatric conditions that may vary in symptomatology but share a common essence. Both of these well-developed models offer deeper insights into the formulation of patients with chronic pain and depression but more importantly make explicit how specific interventions could facilitate rehabilitation.

Clark and Treisman review the 'Neurobiology of Pain' to introduce the next two papers. While basic scientific advances have demonstrated the complexity of the human body, clinical practice must still contend with complicated syndromes such as complex regional pain syndrome (CRPS) and Gulf War syndrome (GWS). Grabow et al. describe these difficulties in 'Complex Regional Pain Syndrome: Diagnostic Controversies, Psychological Dysfunction, and Emerging Concepts'.

No exact pathophysiology explains the entire presentation of patients with CRPS and these patients exhibit a wide variety of somatic complaints, psychological symptoms, and abnormal illness behaviors. Engel et al. take this discussion to the level of prevention in 'Can We Prevent a Second "Gulf War Syndrome"? Population-Based Healthcare for Chronic Idiopathic Pain and Fatigue after War'. The disability and depression manifested by patients with GWS represent one of the most challenging examples of reinforced illness behavior that extends beyond the individual patient into healthcare systems, the military 'family', and society itself as legislated by the government.

The final three papers discuss issues relating to the use of opioids in the treatment of chronic pain. This controversial practice complicated by concerns about substance abuse and malpractice represents another behavioral form of depression. While the medications have an inherent potential for intoxication and abuse, they often reinforce disability through subtle reinforcement that culminates in the depression of dependency on comfort instead of the satisfaction with overcoming challenges. Christo et al. review the use of opioids in 'Opioid Effectiveness, Addiction, and Depression in Chronic Pain'. Olsen and Daumit discuss the problems and expertise required for primary care physicians in 'Opioid Prescribing for Chronic Nonmalignant Pain in Primary Care: Challenges and Solutions'. Geppert expands these topics in 'To Help and Not to Harm: Ethical Issues in the Treatment of Chronic Pain in Patients with Substance Use Disorders'. This special population of patients illuminates the issues discussed throughout this volume for all patients with chronic pain. Physicians, psychiatrists in particular, have an obligation to care for the entire patient. Treatment should restore them to healthy individuals, be mindful of the many ways in which they can be harmed, and employ a formulation of their distress, disability, and depression that extends beyond the algorithms, symptom-based, and homogeneous treatment plans of today's pain centers.

The goal of this volume is to focus the discussion about a complicated problem into complementary domains with concrete examples. Hopefully, this will generate interest and some controversy that will take the conversation about and study of these patients to a new level that will improve the practice of medicine and our patients' outcomes.

*Michael R. Clark*, MD, MPH
*Glenn J. Treisman*, MD, PhD

Clark MR, Treisman GJ (eds): Pain and Depression. An Interdisciplinary Patient-Centered
Approach. Adv Psychosom Med. Basel, Karger, 2004, vol 25, pp 1–27

..........................

# Perspectives on Pain and Depression

*Michael R. Clark*[a], *Glenn J. Treisman*[b]

[a]Chronic Pain Treatment Programs and [b]AIDS Psychiatry Services,
Department of Psychiatry and Behavioral Sciences, Johns Hopkins Medical
Institutions, Baltimore, Md., USA

## Abstract

The health care system is often unsuccessful in the treatment of the patient experiencing
chronic pain. Chronic pain is often complicated by a variety of psychiatric conditions that
make it difficult to engage and treat patients. This generates frustration and pessimism in
the physician. The patient may be afflicted by the syndrome of an affective disorder,
demoralized by the unintended circumstances of their life, unable to meet the demands of
stressors because of a lack of inherent capacities, or helplessly trapped by poor choices
and repeated unproductive actions. The physician's interest and the patient's optimism can
be restored and sustained by utilizing a systematic interdisciplinary approach utilizing the
four perspectives of diseases, life stories, dimensions, and behaviors to evaluate the
patient who is disabled by depression and chronic pain. The design of a comprehensive
treatment plan involves the determination of each perspective's contribution to the
patient's suffering. The process of formulation recognizes that the perspectives are distinct
from one another but complementary in illuminating the various reasons for a patient's
suffering. The perspectives offer a recipe for designing a rational treatment plan rather
than trying to reduce the individual patient's complexity into a one-dimensional construct. This approach increases the probability of a successful outcome for both patient
and physician.

pain (pān) *n* 1: physical suffering typically from injury or illness. 2: distressing
sensation in a part of the body. 3: severe mental or emotional distress. 4: annoying or
troublesome thing

depression, de·pres·sion (di presh'/n) *n* 1: sadness; gloom; dejection. 2: condition
of general emotional dejection and withdrawal; sadness greater and more prolonged
than that warranted by any objective reason. 3: low state of functional activity. 4: dullness
or inactivity

(adapted from Webster's Dictionary, Random House)

## Introduction

The prevalence of chronic pain reported in the general population ranges from 10 to 55% with an estimate of severe chronic pain of approximately 11% among adults despite the lack of standard definitions for terms such as 'chronic' or 'severe' that usually emphasize widespread pain, functional disability, interference from pain, or pain characteristics [Karlsten and Gordh, 1997; Nickel and Raspe, 2001; Ospina and Harstall, 2002; Verhaak et al., 1998]. In the most recent review from multiple countries and the WHO, the weighted mean prevalence of chronic pain was 31% in men, 40% in women, 25% in children up to 18 years old, and 50% in the elderly over 65 years old [Ospina and Harstall, 2002]. During a 2-week period, 13% of the US workforce reported a loss in productivity due to a common pain condition such as headache, back pain, arthritis pain, or other musculoskeletal pain [Stewart et al., 2003].

The US Center for Health Statistics' 8-year follow-up survey found 32.8% of the general population suffered from chronic pain symptoms [Magni et al., 1993]. In another WHO study of over 25,000 primary care patients in 14 countries, 22% (United States = 17%) of patients suffered from pain that was present for most of the time for at least 6 months [Gureje et al., 1998]. In a study of 6,500 individuals aged 15–74 years in Finland, 14% experienced daily chronic pain that was independently associated with lower self-rated health [Mantyselka et al., 2003]. A retrospective analysis of 14,000 primary care patients in Sweden found that approximately 30% of patients seeking treatment had some kind of defined pain problem with almost two thirds diagnosed with musculoskeletal pain [Hasselstrom et al., 2002].

## Types of Pain and Depression

Pain is a complex experience that is influenced by affective, cognitive, and behavioral factors, and has an extensive neurobiology [Meldrum, 2003; Turk et al., 1983]. Pain has been defined by the International Association for the Study of Pain as 'an unpleasant sensory and emotional experience associated with actual or potential tissue damage, or described in terms of such damage' [Merskey et al., 1986]. Chronic pain can be described both by pathophysiological mechanism and anatomical location. For example, peripheral pain can be caused by injury to terminal nerve receptor fields or disrupted integration at peripheral synapses. In contrast, central pain may be related to dysfunctional integration in the spinal cord, brainstem, or higher cortical structures. Pain has sensory, autonomic afferent, and efferent components. The patient with chronic pain will respond differently to interventions depending on the type of pain pathophysiology. A comprehensive evaluation should assess initiating, sustaining, and comorbid factors contributing to their condition [Clark, 2000; Clark and Cox, 2002]. For the purposes of the discussion here, we will presume that physiological factors that cause and exacerbate pain have been evaluated and adequately addressed.

Patients' experiences of suffering, their language and behaviors, and the neurobiological conception of nociception all support a psychological component of pain [Hunt and Mantyh, 2001; Price, 2000]. Cross-sectional studies have consistently found an association between chronic pain and psychological distress, often referred to as 'depression' [Wilson et al., 2001]. In a sample of over 3,000 individuals, psychiatric disorder was a significant predictor of new onset physical symptoms such as back, chest, and abdominal pain 7 years after evaluation [Hotopf et al., 1998]. In a population-based case-control study, the prevalence of a mental disorder was more than 3 times higher in patients with chronic widespread pain than in those without such pain [Benjamin et al., 2000]. Sixty-five percent of patients hospitalized for rehabilitation for a musculoskeletal disease had a lifetime history of a psychiatric disorder [Harter et al., 2002]. Over 30% of patients met criteria for a current mental disorder (11% major depression) with half having two or more psychiatric conditions. In patients with chronic pain, depression occurs for many reasons. The formulation of a patient's case attempts to refine their experience of depression into the dysphoria of an affective disorder, the demoralization of their life circumstances, the distress of being ill-equipped to cope with specific demands, or the disappointment with the consequences of their own actions.

### Chronic Pain Treatment Goals

The goal of treating patients with chronic pain is still the subject of debate. Some feel strongly that the compassionate physician has a duty to prevent suffering, and to that end, the goal of treatment is to eliminate pain as completely as possible regardless the sacrifices. Others feel that patients suffer when they are impaired in their function and that the ultimate goals of treatment should be improving function, longevity, and quality of life. Patients with chronic pain often become more disabled in the pursuit of the goal of comfort. This leads to increases in chronic pain. As an example, diminished mobility leads to the use of a wheelchair, which in turn leads to worsening back and leg pain, obesity, and further diminishment of mobility.

The approach to these patients should emphasize rehabilitation with improvement in function and restoration of health. While treatment outcome studies are positive, many patients with chronic pain are refractory to treatment, continue to suffer, and remain disabled. Many psychiatric barriers to treatment have been

**Table 1.** Summary of the perspectives of psychiatry

|  | Life stories | Behaviors | Dimensions | Diseases |
|---|---|---|---|---|
| Logic | accumulated events produce a unique personal narrative | actions have an underlying design and purpose | personal features are quantified along spectrums of measurement | causal relationships define categorical diagnoses |
| Essence | meaningful connections between past events and present circumstances | goal-directed behaviors require choice and free will | relative amounts of a trait predispose to inherent strengths and vulnerabilities | abnormal structure or function of a bodily part |
| Goal | restore mastery | restore productivity | restore emotional stability | restore function |
| Means | understand patterns, appreciate circumstances, and reinterpret meaning | stop behavior, alter drives/goals, emphasize responsibility and relapse prevention | guide toward settings that evoke strengths and avoid provocation of vulnerabilities | prevent, correct, or palliate the abnormality |

identified and include depression, personality traits, behavioral disruptions, and personal experiences and beliefs. The formulation of chronic pain simply as a symptom of a disease of the body fails to appreciate the role of these factors and results in poor treatment outcome. The complexity of these conditions requires a more comprehensive formulation than the biomedical paradigm can provide.

**Formulation of Depression**

If patients with chronic pain are going to benefit from treatment, a systematic approach that produces a comprehensive formulation and leads to an individualized treatment plan needs to be made explicit [McHugh, 1987, 1992]. The fundamental reasons for the patient's suffering must be specified and can be organized utilizing four perspectives: diseases, life stories, dimensions, and behaviors [McHugh and Slavney, 1982, 1998]. Each perspective offers its own essential logic and method of reasoning beginning with the meaningful circumstances of the patient's life and progressing to the type of unique person involved, then the choices, actions and behaviors of that person, and finally, ending up with the stereotypic diseases that afflict patients (table 1).

***Table 2.*** Step-by-step approach to the individual patient with chronic pain

---

*Diseases*
Consider that the patient's distress is due to an unrecognized clinical syndrome
Search for all possible broken parts causing pathological processes
Fix as many broken parts as completely as possible to minimize pathology
Select treatments that will minimize new damage and subsequent pathology
Utilize palliative treatments when cures are unavailable

*Life stories*
Expand the history to include every aspect of the patient's life
Understand what it means to the patient to suffer from chronic pain
Determine if the patient's distress is due to events he has encountered
Reinterpret these events to provide new insights
Help the patient find an answer to the question, 'What good does life hold for me?'

*Dimensions*
Obtain descriptions of who the patient was before their illness
Supplement this information with standardized instruments
Quantify the amount of each trait a patient possesses
Identify the specific demands/situations that are evoking the patient's vulnerabilities
Provide new skills for deficient traits and match strengths to new tasks

*Behaviors*
Point out all problematic behaviors that need to stop
Focus on repeated actions that undermine the patient's progress
Insist the patient take responsibility for his choices and recognize their consequences
Emphasize productive behaviors and reinforce any positive change
Expect and plan for relapse

---

In this approach to patient care, diseases are what people *have*; life stories and experiences generate and direct what people want; dimensions are who people are, and behaviors are what people do. The physician should formulate the case of a patient with chronic pain by looking for and thinking about the individual contributions from each perspective to the overall presentation (table 2). A treatment plan that addresses all perspectives can then be designed.

Depression can also be formulated from different perspectives. A large number of factors, their interrelationships, and how they contribute to ongoing suffering and eventually successful treatment must be considered [Keefe et al., 1996; Turk and Okifuji, 2002]. Major depression is best explained as a derangement of biological brain function that produces a syndrome of diminished rewards, mood, self-attitude, and vital sense. This last feature includes a sense of illness, increased sensitivity to pain, a variety of medically unexplained somatic symptoms, and circadian rhythm disruption. Depression can be a direct manifestation of intoxication or withdrawal states produced by various substances.

Depression also describes the sadness and low mood associated with psychological adversity. For the purposes of our discussion, the term demoralization describes the broad spectrum of grief, mourning, disappointment, sadness, and loss associated with the circumstances of living with chronic pain and medical illness. Depression also is associated with certain types of personality traits such as pessimism, dissatisfaction, or anxiety. Lastly, depression can be the product of state-dependent learning that is an entrained outcome of certain illness behaviors.

While individuals can be affected by their experiences in the external world and their interpretation of it, these interpretations are shaped by their own drives, traits, and beliefs. They make decisions about their suffering and take purposeful actions to express their distress. The physician's initial role in the evaluation of a patient with chronic pain is to produce a comprehensive formulation and a differential diagnosis attempting to sort out to what extent the patient is demoralized by a particular sequence of meaningful events, frustrated by his own psychological trait vulnerabilities, upset by the consequences of repeatedly choosing to engage in problematic behaviors, or sick with a specific disease [Clark, 1994, 1996; Clark and Swartz, 2001]. Tailoring interventions to patient profiles based on a comprehensive formulation will improve outcome.

### Diseases (table 1)

The disease perspective utilizes the logic of categories of pathology. The disease perspective assumes an abnormality in the structure or function of a bodily part that 'breaks' individuals. The broken part predictably transforms normal physiology into syndromal pathophysiology. Sickness replaces health. As a consequence, pathological signs and symptoms of the disease emerge and cluster together as a recognizable clinical entity. The patient either has a particular disease or he does not. The disease perspective demands searching for the broken part that results in pain.

For example, a patient with burning pain in a particular dermatome is examined and formulated as having the clinical syndrome of neuropathic pain. Further examination attempts to determine what pathology is present such as demyelination, peripheral sensitization, or central deafferentation. These pathological changes result in syndromal signs and symptoms such as sensory loss, allodynia, and hyperalgesia. The patient may have inflammation, infarction, or compression of the involved peripheral nerve. Each of these pathologies, for example compression, has an associated list of potential etiologies of disease such as a tumor caused by increased cell division, an aneurysm caused by weakened smooth muscle in a blood vessel, or excessive bone formation caused by osteoblast activation. Some mental disorders are best explained as diseases such as dementia, schizophrenia, or major depression.

The Canadian National Population Health Survey found that the incidence of major depression was approximately doubled in subjects who reported a long-term medical condition such as back problems, migraine, and sinusitis [Patten, 2001]. In 1,016 HMO members, the prevalence of depression was 12% in individuals with 3 or more pain complaints compared to only 1% in those with one or no pain complaints [Dworkin et al., 1990]. One third to over 50% of patients presenting to clinics specializing in the evaluation of chronic pain have a current major depression [Dersh et al., 2002; Fishbain et al., 1997b; Reich et al., 1983; Smith, 1992]. In groups of patients with medically unexplained symptoms such as back pain, orofacial pain, and dizziness, two thirds of patients have a history of recurrent major depression, compared to less than 20% of medically ill control groups [Atkinson et al., 1991; Katon and Sullivan, 1990; Sullivan and Katon, 1993; Yap et al., 2002].

Physical symptoms are common in patients suffering from major depression [Lipowski, 1990]. Approximately 60% of patients with depression report pain symptoms at the time of diagnosis [Magni et al., 1985; Von Knorring et al., 1983]. In the WHO's data from 14 countries on five continents, 69% (range 45–95%) of patients with depression presented with only somatic symptoms, of which pain complaints were the most common [Simon et al., 1999]. Half the depressed patients reported multiple unexplained somatic symptoms and 11% actively denied the psychological symptoms of depression. A survey of almost 19,000 Europeans found a 4-fold increase in the prevalence of chronic painful conditions in subjects with major depression [Ohayon and Schatzberg, 2003].

The presence of a depressive disorder has been demonstrated to increase the risk of developing chronic musculoskeletal pain, headache, and chest pain up to 3 years later [Leino and Magni, 1993; Magni et al., 1993, 1994; Von Korff et al., 1993]. Even after 8 years, previously depressed patients remained twice as likely to develop chronic pain as the nondepressed. In a 15-year prospective study of workers in an industrial setting, initial depression symptoms predicted low back pain and a positive clinical back exam in men but not women [Leino and Magni, 1993]. Five years later, self-assessed depression at baseline was a significant predictor in the 25% of at-risk women who developed fibromyalgia [Forseth et al., 1999].

Depression worsens other medical illnesses, interferes with their ongoing management, and amplifies their detrimental effects on health-related quality of life [Cassano and Fava, 2002; Gaynes et al., 2002]. Depression in patients with chronic pain is associated with greater pain intensity, more pain persistence, less life control, more use of passive-avoidant coping strategies, noncompliance with treatment, application for early retirement, and greater interference from pain including more pain behaviors observed by others [Hasenbring et al., 1994; Haythornthwaite et al., 1991; Kerns and Haythornthwaite, 1988; Magni et al., 1985, 1993; Weickgenant et al., 1993]. Primary care patients with musculoskeletal pain complicated by depression are significantly more likely to use medications daily, in combinations, and that include sedative-hypnotics [Mantyselka et al., 2002]. In a study of over 15,000 employees who filed health claims, the cost of managing chronic conditions such as back problems was multiplied by 1.7 when they also suffered from a comorbid depression [Druss et al., 2000]. In a clinical trial of 1,001 depressed patients over age 60 years with arthritis, antidepressants and/or problem-solving oriented psychotherapy not only reduced depressive symptoms but also improved pain, functional status, and quality of life [Lin et al., 2003].

Depression is a better predictor of disability than pain intensity and duration [Rudy et al., 1988]. For example, fibromyalgia patients with depression compared to those without were significantly more likely to live alone, report functional disability, and describe maladaptive thoughts [Okifuji et al., 2000]. A naturalistic follow-up study of patients with chronic pain who had substantial numbers of sick days found that a diagnosis of major depression predicted disability an average of 3.7 years later [Ericsson et al., 2002]. The presence of depression in whiplash patients reduced the insurance claim closure rate by 37% [Cote et al., 2001]. This rate was unaffected even after the insurance system eliminated compensation for pain and suffering. Preoperative major depression in patients undergoing surgery for thoracic outlet syndrome increased the rate of self-reported disability by over 15 times [Axelrod et al., 2001]. In patients with rheumatoid arthritis, depressive symptoms were significantly associated with negative health and functional out-comes as well as increased health services utilization [Katz and Yelin, 1993]. Depression consistently predicted level of functioning, pain severity, pain-related disability, less use of active coping, and more use of passive coping in patients in a university chronic pain inpatient unit [Fisher et al., 2001].

The consequences of depression can be extreme. Patients suffering from chronic pain syndromes including migraine, chronic abdominal pain, and orthopedic pain syndromes report increased rates of suicidal ideation, suicide attempts, and suicide completion [Fishbain, 1999; Fishbain et al., 1991; Magni et al., 1998]. In one study of patients who attempted suicide, 52% suffered from a chronic somatic disease and 21% were taking analgesics on a daily basis for pain [Stenager et al., 1994]. Patients with chronic pain completed suicide at 2–3 times the rate in the general population [Fishbain et al., 1991]. Cancer patients with pain and depression, but not pain alone, were significantly more likely to request assistance in committing suicide as well as actively take steps to end their lives [Emanuel et al., 1996].

The determination whether negative affect represents a diagnosis of major depression as opposed to psychological distress varies widely. Principal-component analyses of the responses of patients with chronic pain on the BDI find three factors consistent with the core criteria of major depression: low mood, impaired self attitude, poor vital sense [Novy et al., 1995; Williams and Richardson, 1993]. In a study comparing separate measures of affective distress, self-reported depressive symptoms, and major depression in patients with chronic pain at a pain clinic, a diagnosis of major depression was determined to be a less sensitive indicator and less important predictor of the chronic pain experience than self-reported depressive symptoms [Geisser et al., 2000]. The presence of depressive symptoms, even without the categorical diagnosis of major depression, is an important comorbidity for patients with chronic pain [Bair et al., 2003]. However, if treatment for depression is to be rationally designed and effective, the specific form of depression must be discovered.

Treatment for a disease involves finding a cure for the pathology and restoring function to premorbid levels. The cure may repair the broken part, prevent the initial damage from occurring, or compensate for the affected physiology. The etiology of major depression is elusive and treatments are currently unable to permanently correct the underlying pathology, however many patients are completely free of depressive symptoms while in treatment with antidepressant medications. Major depression must be distinguished from an expected demoralization and sadness that can be 'understood' as an outcome of suffering with chronic pain. Clearly, patients may have both major depression and demoralization. Because physicians are compassionate and empathize with their patients they may 'understand' the depressive feelings associated with major depression and fail to adequately utilize specific psychological and pharmacological therapies.

**Life Stories** (table 1)

An important component of a person's response to adversity is that person's assumptions about the world. These assumptions are based on experiences and the meaning derived from them. A person who is misused by authority figures such as parents during childhood will have problems successfully interacting with authority figures in adulthood. This may disrupt the trust required in the patient-doctor relationship. More importantly, a person's assumptions about the world will in part direct their experiences in the future. This means that a set of negative experiences occurring at a vulnerable time will be magnified by shaping future experiences. A cycle of negative experience leads to meaningful assumptions that then direct behavior. In the example above, patients who do not trust their physician may act in ways that undermine their relationship with the physician. Physicians may then respond with frustration and disappoint the patient magnifying the difficulty of achieving an effective therapeutic alliance.

As these events accumulate, the patient becomes imbedded in a narrative. This narrative is a tapestry of meaningful connections specific to the individual from which he develops an understanding of his own existence and sets of assumptions about his roles in the world. At times, a person experiences the unintended consequences of past events. When life turns out differently from what was expected, the outcome is demoralization. This distress is due to a perceived loss of mastery over one's life. This loss is not the result of the broken part caused by a disease but of an individual left wanting something better from life.

Evaluation within the domain of life stories involves knowing more of the personal story and appreciating the patient's meaningful understanding of those events. In treatment, the patient is persuaded by the physician to give up his current interpretation of those events for another. A new interpretation is not necessarily a more 'correct' or 'true' interpretation. An infinite number of meanings can be generated for a given set of historical life events. The importance of the new interpretation is that it tries to be useful and restore a sense of mastery for the patient. If the patient can embrace a new understanding of his situation and why it has occurred, he can go forward with a renewed sense of control over his life that now again has the potential for success.

These relationships can be very complex. An example is a patient who in childhood grew up in an extremely authoritarian environment with unreasonable expectations and few rewards for success. The patient was expected to get A's in school and anything less was equivalent to failure. This patient found that illness produced decreased expectations for his performance and was 'rewarded' for circumstances of illness with decreased expectations. As an adult, the patient is perfectionistic and chronically dissatisfied with his own performance. A knee injury made it difficult for him to perform at work and ultimately the patient was encouraged to accept disability to decrease the burden on his employer. This produced a feeling of uselessness and disappointment but the patient was trapped by his handicap. Rehabilitative psychotherapy reframed the performance of overcoming the handicap as a success and rewarded the efforts of physical therapy and vocational rehabilitation as a triumph over the adversity of illness. Ultimately, therapy was able to get the patient to recognize the pattern in his life of illness decreasing distress by lowering self-imposed expectations. The patient was successfully able to return to work with ongoing psychotherapy. Recognizing recurring patterns of events would allow for changes to avoid future circumstances of the same kind and restore the individual's sense of mastery.

The cognitive-behavioral model of chronic pain assumes individual perceptions and evaluations of life experiences affect emotional and behavioral reactions to these experiences [Keefe et al., 1996]. If patients believe pain, depression, and disability are inevitable and uncontrollable, then they will experience more negative affective responses, increased pain, and even more impaired physical and psychosocial functioning. The components of cognitive-behavioral therapy (CBT) such as relaxation, cognitive restructuring, and coping self-statement training interrupt this cycle of disability and enhance operant-behavioral treatment [Turner, 1982a, b; Turner and Chapman, 1982]. Patients are taught to become active participants in the management of their pain through the utilization of methods that minimize distressing thoughts and feelings. Outcome studies of CBT in patients with syndromes ranging from specific painful diseases to vague functional somatoform symptoms have demonstrated significant improvements in pain intensity, pain behaviors, physical symptoms, affective distress, depression, coping, physical functioning, treatment-related and indirect socioeconomic costs, and return to work [Hiller et al., 2003; Keefe et al., 1990a; Kroenke and Swindle, 2000; McCracken and Turk, 2002; Turner, 1982a; Turner and Romano, 1990]. The effectiveness of cognitive behavioral treatments in adults with chronic pain has been documented in a meta-analysis across numerous outcome domains [Morley et al., 1999]. Pain reduction and improved physical function have been found to continue up to 12 months after the completion of active cognitive-behavioral treatment [Gardea et al., 2001; Keefe et al., 1990b; Nielson and Weir, 2001].

Ultimately, the goal of treating patients with chronic pain is to end disability, return people to work or other productive activities, and improve quality of life. Patients with chronic pain encounter many obstacles to return to work including their own negative perceptions and beliefs about work [Grossi et al., 1999; Marhold et al., 2002; Schult et al., 2000]. In a longitudinal follow-up study of chronic back pain, patients who were not working and involved in litigation had the highest scores on measures of pain, depression, and disability [Suter, 2002]. One of the most important predictors is the patient's own intention of returning to work, which is less likely to be a function of pain than job characteristics [Fishbain et al., 1997b]. For example, job availability, satisfaction, dangerousness, physical demands, and litigation status are more likely to influence a patient's return to work [Fishbain et al., 1995, 1999a; Hildebrandt et al., 1997].

Treatment strategies in the life story perspective focus on instilling in the patient a desire for a life that is more fulfilling. The success of CBT has focused attention on many elements of the chronic pain experience to improve outcome. A negative perception of the future by the patient with chronic pain will lead to an increase in distress, a sense of losing social support, and the use of maladaptive coping skills [Hellstrom et al., 1999, 2000]. Adjustment is defined as the ability to carry out normal physical and psychosocial activities. The three dimensions of adjustment are social functioning (e.g., employment, functional ability), morale (e.g., depression, anxiety), and somatic health (e.g., pain intensity, medication use, health care utilization) [Jensen et al., 1991a; Lazarus and Folkman, 1984]. These concepts address resilience to the effects of chronic illness, the alleviation of suffering, and the development of a more positive concept of self or identity for the patient [Buchi et al., 2002]. As an individual reflects on his life, the process of understanding and adjustment should address the meaning of his illness, planning specific interventions to minimize any disability, and finding opportunities to maximize quality of life.

Acceptance of chronic pain is a factor reported to influence patient adjustment. The analysis of patient accounts of their acceptance of chronic pain involved themes such as taking control, living day to day, acknowledging limitations, empowerment, accepting loss of self, believing there is more to life than pain, not fighting battles that cannot be won, and reliance on spiritual strength [Risdon et al., 2003]. Greater acceptance of pain has been associated with a variety of factors including decreased disability and pain-related anxiety [McCracken, 1998]. Self-esteem and social support are factors predictive of improved acceptance of various types of disability [Li and Moore, 1998]. Therefore, acceptance is a realistic approach to living with pain that incorporates both the disengagement from struggling against pain and engagement in productive everyday activities with achievable goals. Achieving acceptance of pain is associated with reports of lower pain intensity, less pain-related anxiety and avoidance, less depression, less physical and psychosocial disability, more daily uptime, and better work status [McCracken, 1998]. Acceptance of pain predicted better overall adjustment to pain and patient functioning [McCracken et al., 1999].

### Dimensions (table 1)

While depression may be both a cause and a consequence of chronic pain, there are mediating factors in the complex relationship [Banks and Kerns, 1996; Fishbain et al., 1997a; Pincus and Williams, 1999; Sheftell and Atlas, 2002]. The diathesis-stress model postulates an interaction between personal premorbid vulnerabilities activated and exacerbated by life stressors such as chronic pain with the subsequent outcome of depression or other psychopathology. The dimensional perspective is based on the logic of a continuous distribution of individual variation. Traits are personal characteristics and bodily processes that can be quantified along a continuum or distribution of measurement. Traits are the elements that make people who they are. Most individuals possess an average amount of a particular trait; however, a few individuals will have very little or excessive amounts. The trait itself conveys an ability that becomes an asset in one set of circumstances or a liability in another. The inherent strengths and weaknesses of the individual vary depending on the individual 'dose' of the characteristic and the task at hand that places specific demands upon the person. Problems occur when patients encounter a high frequency of circumstances for which they are poorly adapted due to their inherent traits.

Traits involve potentials and not destinies. Standardized assessments of traits can provide efficient and detailed information about an individual. However, no one instrument has proven comprehensive and relevant for all patients with chronic pain. Treatments within the dimensional perspective focus on emphasizing the strengths and weaknesses that are the manifestations of particular characteristics and the settings that evoke them such as being anxious in unfamiliar situations. Specific methods must be devised to compensate for the individual patient's vulnerabilities such as providing vocational training. With guidance and new skills, success can be achieved by seeking out situations that are a better match to the person's specific trait composition and capable of evoking his strengths.

An example of a dimensional trait is found in the domain of affective temperament. Several studies have focused on the personality characteristics and disorders of patients with chronic pain [Vendrig et al., 2000; Weisberg, 2000; Weisberg and Vaillancourt, 1999]. Previous studies have identified Minnesota Multiphasic Personality Inventory (MMPI) cluster profiles such as the conversion 'V' type and neurotic triad with different multivariate relationships between other constructs such as somatization, coping strategies, depression, pain severity, and activity level [Riley and Robinson, 1998]. However, while patients with chronic pain differ from nonchronic pain controls in their scale profiles on the MMPI, there is no single personality type associated with medically unexplained chronic pain or chronic pain from 'organic' diseases. Personality traits should be appreciated as sustaining or modifying factors that have the potential to complicate the treatment process rather than as causes of or the sole explanation for chronic pain [Vendrig, 2000]. The personality vulnerabilities, therefore, contribute to the degree of potential disability that individuals experience by modifying their response to pain.

An example is a patient presenting with suicidal feelings in the context of chronic pain, disability, and benzodiazepine abuse. The patient was injured when a bus she was riding collided with another vehicle resulting in a facial injury. She was mildly disfigured and had chronic jaw pain exacerbated by chewing and talking. The patient described herself as always seeing the glass half empty and being depressed her whole life. Despite this, she had been functional, working full time, and successful in her marriage prior to her injury. She admitted that she believed her spouse no longer found her attractive and had withdrawn from an intimate life with him. Her job required frequent public speaking and contact with clients. Her anxiety about her appearance and speech incapacitated her. A series of meetings with her previous employer and husband allowed the treatment team to confront her about the manner in which her personality was sabotaging her rehabilitation. It also allowed the treatment team to describe how much more empty her glass would be if she did not recover. Ultimately, she was able to return to work and reestablish her marital relationship. She was extremely difficult to taper from benzodiazepines because of her trait anxiety that was exacerbated by withdrawal. Inpatient treatment was able to provide the necessary support and encouragement to successfully complete the taper.

Coping has been defined as 'a person's cognitive and behavioral efforts to manage the internal and external demands of the person-environment transaction that is appraised as taxing or exceeding the person's resources' [Folkmanet al., 1986; Jensen et al., 1991a]. Higher levels of disability were found in persons who remain passive or use coping strategies of catastrophizing, ignoring or reinterpreting pain sensations, diverting attention from pain, and praying or hoping for relief. In a 6-month follow-up study of patients completing an inpatient pain program, improvement was associated with decreases in the use of passive coping strategies [Jensen et al., 1994]. Negative self-statements have been found to be predictive of general activity, pain interference, and affective distress [Stroud et al., 2000]. The transtheoretical model of change proposes that patients progress through specific stages as their readiness to adopt new beliefs increases and subsequent coping skills improve [Jensen et al., 2000; Kerns et al., 1997].

The effectiveness of particular coping strategies is dependent on many aspects of a patient's experience with chronic pain [Tan et al., 2001]. Higher levels of pain-related anxiety are associated with greater pain severity, interference of pain, and difficulty with daily activities in men but *not* women with chronic pain [Edwards et al., 2000]. Patients with fibromyalgia compared to work-related muscular pain reported higher levels of trait anxiety and pain-related catastrophizing and low levels of abilities to control and reduce pain [Hallberg and Carlsson, 1998]. Catastrophic thinking about pain has been attributed to the amplification of threatening information and it interferes with the focus needed to facilitate patients remaining involved with productive instead of pain-related activities [Crombez et al., 1998]. Catastrophizing intensifies the experience of pain and increases emotional distress as well as self-perceived disability [Severeijns et al., 2001; Sullivan et al., 2001]. This multidimensional construct includes elements of cognitive rumination, symptom magnification, and feelings of helplessness [Van Damme et al., 2002].

Pain-related cognitive traits like catastrophizing are considered some of the strongest psychological variables mediating the transition from acute to chronic pain and usually have more predictive power of poor adjustment to chronic pain than objective factors such as disease status, physical impairment, or occupational descriptions [Hasenbring et al., 2001]. In a population-based study of individuals without low back pain, high levels of catastrophizing and fear of injury prospectively predicted disability due to new onset low back pain 6 months later [Picavet et al., 2002]. In a study of patients with pain after spinal cord injury, catastrophizing was associated with poor adjustment [Turner et al., 2002]. Dispositional optimism is an intrinsic personal feature that affects types of coping with chronic pain [Novy et al., 1998]. Optimism as well as other traits increase the ability of patients to find benefits from living with adversity such as major medical problems like chronic pain [Affleck and Tennen, 1996].

Treatment within the dimensional perspective identifies the demands that are evoking the patient's vulnerabilities, focusing on enhancing the deficient traits, and finding new situations that will capitalize on the patient's strengths. For example, pain-related fear and catastrophizing of patients improved more when they were exposed in vivo to individually tailored, fear-eliciting, and hier-archically ordered physical movements instead of following a general graded activity treatment program for back pain [Vlaeyen et al., 2002]. Early-treatment catastrophizing and helplessness of patients in a 4-week multidisciplinary pain program predicted late-treatment outcomes such as pain-related interference and activity level [Burns et al., 2003]. These changes persisted despite controlling for changes in depression over the course of treatment, supporting the model that changing negative cognitions improves treatment outcome.

## Behaviors (table 1)

Behaviors are goal-directed activities. Internally, behaviors are motivated by drives such as hunger or seeking relief from pain. These drives provoke the behavior and then abate after some action is performed that satisfies the drive, which then will likely reemerge at some time in the future. Externally, behaviors are meaningful because of the opportunities, self-imposed beliefs, and individual goals that lead to a person making choices. Similarly, behavior has external consequences that are reinforcing to the individual and involve learning over time how to accomplish one's goals more effectively. A self-efficacy expectancy is a belief about one's ability to perform a specific behavior while an outcome expectancy is a belief about the consequences of performing a behavior [Jensen et al., 1991b]. Individuals are considered more likely to engage in actions they believe are both within their capabilities and will result in a positive outcome. Self-efficacy beliefs mediate the relationship between pain intensity and disability in different groups of patients with chronic pain [Arnstein et al., 1999; Arnstein, 2000; Rudy et al., 2003; Turner et al., 2000]. The lack of belief in one's own ability to manage pain, cope and function despite persistent pain is a significant predictor of disability and secondary depression in patients with chronic pain. Patients with a variety of chronic pain syndromes who score higher on measures of self-efficacy report lower levels of pain, higher pain thresholds, increased exercise performance and more positive coping efforts [Asghari and Nicholas, 2001; Barry et al., 2003; Berkke et al., 2001; Lackner and Carosella, 1999].

More sophisticated models of pain and depression add the component of illness behavior (functional disability), which functions both as a response of the vulnerable individual to a significant stressor but then later as a stressor itself [Revenson and Felton, 1989]. The severity of depression has been found to be unaffected by pain intensity when pain-related disability is controlled [Von Korff et al., 1992]. If pain causes disability such as loss of independence or mobility that decreases an individual's participation in activities, the risk of depression is significantly increased [Williamson and Schulz, 1992]. In a clinical trial of patients with chronic low back pain, the association between pain and depression was attributable to disability and illness attitudes [Dickens et al., 2000].

The fear-avoidance model and expectancy model of fear provide explanations for the initiation and maintenance of chronic pain disability with avoidance of specific activities [Greenberg and Burns, 2003; Lethem et al., 1983; Reis, 1991; Vlaeyen and Linton, 2000]. Fear of pain, movement, reinjury, and other negative consequences that result in the avoidance of activities promote the transition to and sustaining of chronic pain and its associated disabilities such as muscular reactivity, deconditioning, and guarded movement [Asmundson et al., 1999]. Patients with chronic low back pain who restricted their activities developed physiological changes (muscle atrophy, osteoporosis, weight gain) and functional deterioration attributed to deconditioning [Verbunt et al., 2003]. This process is reinforced by negative cognitions such as low self-efficacy, catastrophic interpretations, and increased expectations of failure regarding attempts to engage in rehabilitation.

Fear-avoidance beliefs have been found to be one of the most significant predictors of failure to return to work in patients with chronic low back pain [Waddell et al., 1993]. Operant conditioning reinforces disability if the avoidance provides any short-term benefits such as reducing anticipatory anxiety or relieving the patient of unwanted responsibilities. In a study of patients with chronic low back pain, improvements in disability following physical therapy were associated with decreases in pain, psychological distress, and fear-avoidance beliefs but not specific physical deficits [Mannion et al., 1999, 2001]. Decreasing work-specific fears was a more important outcome than addressing general fears of physical activity in predicting improved physical capability for work among patients participating in an interdisciplinary treatment program [Vowles and Gross, 2003]. Patients may require disability status in order to obtain resources needed for rehabilitation and recovery from illness. Unfortunately, improved functional status becomes linked to withdrawal of financial resources. Suddenly, the patients in the midst of rehabilitation find themselves unable to pay for medications or other necessary therapies because their functional status has improved but not completely returned to premorbid levels. Disability resources now reward illness behaviors and undermine recovery. The insurance industry has further complicated this problem by excluding preexisting conditions so that patients who choose to return to work risk losing their disability coverage for the future.

Psychological treatment for chronic pain was pioneered by Fordyce et al. [1973] using an operant conditioning behavioral model. The behavioral approach is based on an understanding of pain in a social context. The behaviors of the patient with chronic pain not only reinforce the behaviors of others but also are reinforced by others. Therapies for behavioral disorders have focused on modifying drives and reinforcements to stop problematic actions such as pain behaviors, medication use, and excessive utilization of health care services. Pain behaviors such as grimacing, guarding, and taking pain medication are indicators of perceived pain severity and functional disability [Chapman et al., 1985; Fordyce et al., 1984; Keefe et al., 1986; Romano et al., 1988; Turk and Matyas, 1992; Turk and Okifuji, 1997]. Behavioral treatments promote the adaptation of a person to their pain by encouraging healthy, productive actions.

Active physical therapy is a specific form of behavior therapy directed at reducing pain behaviors by increasing muscle strength and endurance as well as altering abnormal body mechanics that have developed to compensate for a specific dysfunction. This behavioral rehabilitation involves performing a series of exercises and implementing postural changes with the goals of recovering normal functional capacity throughout the body. These exercises also have a psychological benefit as patients learn to take an active role in a treatment that increases their functional capacity [Yardley and Luxon, 1994]. Patients on sick leave with nonspecific low back pain treated with the addition of problem-solving therapy to behavioral graded activity had significantly fewer future sick leave days, higher rates of returning to work, and lower rates of receiving disability pensions [Van den Hout et al., 2003].

Aberrant drug taking behavior represents a specialized subgroup of behavioral disorders. In most people, aberrant behaviors are suppressed when they begin to interfere with productive functioning. Patients with chronic pain, depression, personality vulnerabilities, and demoralization are at increased risk for developing excessive self-administration of reinforcing medications. The ways in which medications reinforce these patients include both direct reward-producing effects as well as the relief of both pain and depression.

The prevalence of substance use disorders in patients with chronic pain is higher than in the general population [Dersh et al., 2002; Weaver and Schnoll, 2002]. In a study of primary care outpatients with chronic noncancer pain who received at least 6 months of opioid prescriptions during 1 year, behaviors consistent with opioid abuse were recorded in approximately 25% of patients [Reid et al., 2002]. Almost 90% of patients attending a pain management clinic were taking medications and 70% were prescribed opioid analgesics [Kouyanou et al., 1997]. In this population, 12% met DSM-III-R criteria for substance abuse or dependence. In another study of 414 chronic pain patients, 23% met criteria for active alcohol, opioid, or sedative misuse or dependency, 9% met criteria for a remission diagnosis, and current dependency was most common for opioids (13%) [Hoffman et al., 1995]. In reviews of substance dependence or addiction in patients with chronic pain, the prevalence ranges from 3 to 19% in high quality studies [Fishbain et al., 1992; Nicholson, 2003].

Recent efforts have attempted to standardize diagnostic criteria and definitions for problematic medication use behaviors and substance use disorders across professional disciplines (table 2) [American Academy of Pain Medicine, 2001; Chabal et al., 1997; Greenwald et al., 1999; Savage, 2002]. The core criteria for a substance use disorder in patients with chronic pain include the loss of control in the use of the medication, excessive preoccupation with it despite adequate analgesia, and adverse consequences associated with its use [Compton et al., 1998]. Items from the Prescription Drug Use Questionnaire that best predicted the presence of addiction in a sample of patients with problematic medication use were (1) the patients believing they were addicted, (2) increasing analgesic dose/frequency, and (3) a preferred route of administration. The presence of maladaptive behaviors must be demonstrated to diagnose addiction.

Determining whether patients with chronic pain are abusing prescribed controlled substances is a routine but challenging issue in care [Miotto et al., 1996; Compton et al., 1998; Robinson et al., 2001; Savage, 2002]. In one survey of approximately 12,000 medical inpatients treated with opioids for a variety of conditions drawn from the Boston Collaborative Drug Surveillance Program, only 4 patients without a history of substance abuse were reported to have developed dependence on the medication [Porter and Jick, 1980]. While this report was based on a large sample and extensive medication database, the methods were not detailed and specifically did not describe the criteria for addiction or the extent of follow-up performed. Other studies of opioid therapy have found that patients who developed problems with their medication all had a history of substance abuse [Portenoy and Foley, 1986; Taub, 1982]. However, inaccurate and underreporting of medication use by patients complicates assessment [Fishbain et al., 1999b; Ready et al., 1982]. Not infrequently, prior substance abuse history emerges only after current misuse has been identified, thus requiring physicians to be vigilant over the course of treatment. In patients with chronic pain who did develop new substance use disorders, the problem most commonly involved the medications prescribed by their physicians [Long et al., 1988; Maruta et al., 1979].

The causes and onset of substance use disorders have been difficult to characterize in relationship to chronic pain. During the first 5 years after the onset of chronic pain, patients are at increased risk for developing new substance use disorders and additional physical injuries [Brown et al., 1996; Savage, 1993]. A cycle of pain followed by relief after taking medications is a classic example of operant reinforcement of future medication use that eventually becomes abuse [Fordyce et al., 1973]. Drug-seeking behavior may be the result of a depressed patient trying to achieve or maintain a previous level of pain control. In this situation, the patient's actions likely represent pseudoaddiction that results from therapeutic dependence and current or potential undertreatment but not addiction [Kirsh et al., 2002; Weaver and Schnoll, 2002].


### Conclusion

Chronic pain is exacerbated by comorbid depression, and depression is exacerbated by chronic pain. There is ample evidence that both conditions are underrecognized and undertreated. It is also clear that both problems pose significant public health problems and associated with enormous financial costs. There is accumulating evidence that the cost of treatment is trivial compared to the cost of ongoing disability and suffering. Specialty recognition of the inter-action between these two conditions and the development of comprehensive treatment plans involving multiple specialists are imperative. Unfortunately, in the climate of cost containment and fiscal responsibility over the short term, the long-term costs of these problems have accelerated with the closure of programs specifically designed to care for these patients. All physicians must advocate for better care of these patients but the provision of interdisciplinary specialty clinics that can formulate cases with the complexities described must be provided and funded.

Each perspective of an interdisciplinary formulation has a unique logic that defines specific methods for designing treatment for the patient with depression and chronic pain. The patient does not have to fit into one theoretical approach or model in order to receive and accept treatment. The patient's treatment is based on the formulation, which becomes rational instead of programmatic. The linkages and interactions of a patient's diagnoses can then be investigated within a framework that includes the entire person and not just their biochemistry.

If a patient's suffering persists, other factors must be considered that may have been overlooked before the treatment plan is abandoned or modified. Usually these factors are within one of the perspectives initially thought to be less important. A new combination of approaches is then required to treat the patient successfully. The perspectives appreciate that the patient is struggling through important life events, but also that he is a person composed of vulnerabilities and strengths, having made many choices, and afflicted by diseases.

## References

Affleck G, Tennen H: Construing benefits from adversity: Adaptational significance and dispositional underpinnings. J Pers 1996;64:899–922.

American Academy of Pain Medicine, the American Pain Society and the American Society of Addiction Medicine: Definitions related to the use of opioids for the treatment of pain. WMJ 2001;100: 28–29.

Arnstein P: The mediation of disability by self efficacy in different samples of chronic pain patients. Disabil Rehabil 2000;22:794–801.

Arnstein P, Caudill M, Mandle CL, et al: Self efficacy as a mediator of the relationship between pain intensity, disability and depression in chronic pain patients. Pain 1999;80:483–491.

Asghari A, Nicholas MK: Pain self-efficacy beliefs and pain behaviour. A prospective study. Pain 2001;94:85–100.

Asmundson GJG, Norton PJ, Norton GR: Beyond pain: The role of fear and avoidance in chronicity. Clin Psychol Rev 1999;19:97–119.

Atkinson JH, Slater MA, Patterson TL, et al: Prevalence, onset and risk of psychiatric disorders in men with chronic low back pain: A controlled study. Pain 1991;45:111–121.

Axelrod DA, Proctor MC, Geisser ME, et al: Outcomes after surgery for thoracic outlet syndrome. J Vasc Surg 2001;33:1220–1225.

Bair MJ, Robinson RL, Katon W, et al: Depression and pain comorbidity: A literature review. Arch Intern Med 2003;163:2433–2445.

Banks SM, Kerns RD: Explaining high rates of depression in chronic pain: A diathesis-stress framework. Psychol Bull 1996;199:95–110.

Barry LC, Guo Z, Kerns RD, et al: Functional self-efficacy and pain-related disability among older veterans with chronic pain in a primary care setting. Pain 2003;104:131–137.

Benjamin S, Morris S, McBeth J, et al: The association between chronic widespread pain and mental disorder: A population-based study. Arthritis Rheum 2000;43:561–567.

Berkke M, Hjortdahl P, Kvien TK: Involvement and satisfaction: A Norwegian study of health care among 1,024 patients with rheumatoid arthritis and 1,509 patients with chronic noninflammatory musculoskeletal pain. Arthritis Rheum 2001;45:8–15.

Brown RL, Patterson JJ, Rounds LA, et al: Substance use among patients with chronic pain. J Fam Pract 1996;43:152–160.

Buchi S, Buddeberg C, Klaghofer R, et al: Preliminary validation of PRISM (Pictorial Representation of Illness and Self Measure) – A brief method to assess suffering. Psychother Psychosom 2002;71: 333–341.

Burns JW, Kubilus A, Bruehl S, et al: Do changes in cognitive factors influence outcome following multidisciplinary treatment for chronic pain? A cross-lagged panel analysis. J Consult Clin Psychol 2003;71:81–91.

Cassano P, Fava M: Depression and public health: An overview. J Psychosom Res 2002;53:849–857.

Chabal C, Erjavec MK, Jacobson L, et al: Prescription opiate abuse in chronic pain patients: Clinical criteria, incidence, and predictors. Clin J Pain 1997;13:150–155.

Chapman CR, Casey KL, Dubner R, et al: Pain measurement: An overview. Pain 1985;22:1–31.

Clark MR: Chronic dizziness: An integrated approach. Hosp Pract 1994;29:57–64.

Clark MR: The role of psychiatry in the treatment of chronic pain; in Campbell J, Cohen M (eds): Pain Treatment Centers at a Crossroads: A Practical and Conceptual Reappraisal. Seattle, IASP Press, 1996, pp 59–68.

Clark MR: Pain; in Coffey CE, Cummings JL (eds): Textbook of Geriatric Neuropsychiatry. Washington, American Psychiatric Press, 2000, pp 415–440.

Clark MR, Cox TS: Refractory chronic pain. Psychiatr Clin North Am 2002;25:71–88.

Clark MR, Swartz KL: A conceptual structure and methodology for the systematic approach to the evaluation and treatment of patients with chronic dizziness. J Anxiety Disord 2001;15:95–106.

Compton P, Darakjian J, Miotto K: Screening for addiction in patients with chronic pain and 'problematic' substance use: Evaluation of a pilot assessment tool. J Pain Symptom Manage 1998;16: 355–363.

Cote P, Hogg-Johnson S, Cassidy JD, et al: The association between neck pain intensity, physical functioning, depressive symptomatology and time-to-claim-closure after whiplash. J Clin Epidemiol 2001;54:275–286.

Crombez G, Eccleston C, Baeyens F, et al: When somatic information threatens, catastrophic thinking enhances attentional interference. Pain 1998;75:187–198.

Dersh J, Polatin PB, Gatchel RJ: Chronic pain and psychopathology: Research findings and theoretical considerations. Psychosom Med 2002;64:773–786.

Dickens C, Jayson M, Sutton C, et al: The relationship between pain and depression in a trial using paroxetine in sufferers of chronic low back pain. Psychosomatics 2000;41:490–499.

Druss BG, Rosenheck RA, Sledge WH: Health and disability costs of depressive illness in a major U.S. corporation. Am J Psychiatry 2000;157:1274–1278.

Dworkin SF, Von Korff M, LeResche L: Multiple pains and psychiatric disturbance: An epidemiologic investigation. Arch Gen Psychiatry 1990;47:239–244.

Edwards R, Augustson EM, Fillingim R: Sex-specific effects of pain-related anxiety on adjustment to chronic pain. Clin J Pain 2000;16:46–53.

Emanuel EJ, Fairclough DL, Daniels ER, et al: Euthanasia and physician-assisted suicide: Attitudes and experiences of oncology patients, oncologists, and the public. Lancet 1996;347:1805–1810.

Ericsson M, Poston WS, Linder J, et al: Depression predicts disability in long-term chronic pain patients. Disabil Rehabil 2002;24:334–340.

Fishbain DA: The association of chronic pain and suicide. Semin Clin Neuropsychiatry 1999;4:221–227.

Fishbain DA, Cutler RB, Rosomoff HL, et al: Chronic pain-associated depression: Antecedent or consequence of chronic pain? A review. Clin J Pain 1997a;13:116–137.

Fishbain DA, Cutler RB, Rosomoff HL, et al: Impact of chronic pain patients' job perception variables on actual return to work. Clin J Pain 1997b;13:197–206.

Fishbain DA, Cutler RB, Rosomoff HL, et al: Prediction of 'intent', 'discrepancy with intent', and 'discrepancy with nonintent' for the patient with chronic pain to return to work after treatment at a pain facility. Clin J Pain 1999a;15:141–150.

Fishbain DA, Cutler RB, Rosomoff HL, et al: Validity of self-report drug use in chronic pain patients. Clin J Pain 1999b;15:184–191.

Fishbain DA, Goldberg M, Rosomoff RS, et al: Completed suicide in chronic pain. Clin J Pain 1991;7: 29–36.

---

Fishbain DA, Rosomoff HL, Cutler RB, et al: Do chronic pain patients' perceptions about their preinjury jobs determine their intent to return to the same type of job post-pain facility treatment. Clin J Pain 1995;11:267–278.

Fishbain DA, Rosomoff HL, Rosomoff RS: Drug abuse, dependence: Addiction in chronic pain patients. Clin J Pain 1992;8:77–85.

Fisher BJ, Haythornthwaite JA, Heinberg LJ, et al: Suicidal intent in patients with chronic pain. Pain 2001;89:199–206.

Folkman S, Lazarus RS, Gruen RJ, et al: Appraisal, coping, health status, and psychological symptoms. J Pers Soc Psychol 1986;50:571–579.

Fordyce W, Fowler R, Lehmann J, et al: Operant conditioning in the treatment of chronic pain. Arch Phys Med Rehabil 1973;54:399–408.

Fordyce WE, Lansky D, Calsyn DA, et al: Pain measurement and pain behavior. Pain 1984;18:53–69.

Forseth KO, Husby G, Gran JT, et al: Prognostic factors for the development of fibromyalgia in women with self-reported musculoskeletal pain. A prospective study. J Rheumatol 1999;26:2458–2467.

Gardea MA, Gatchel RJ, Mishra KD: Long-term efficacy of biobehavioral treatment of temporomandibular disorders. J Behav Med 2001;24:341–359.

Gaynes BN, Burns BJ, Tweed DL, et al: Depression and health-related quality of life. J Nerv Ment Dis 2002;190:799–806.

Geisser ME, Roth RS, Theisen ME, et al: Negative affect, self-report of depressive symptoms, and clinical depression: Relation to the experience of chronic pain. Clin J Pain 2000;16:110–120.

Greenberg J, Burns JW: Pain anxiety among chronic pain patients: Specific phobia or manifestation of anxiety sensitivity? Behav Res Ther 2003;41:223–240.

Greenwald BD, Narcessian EJ, Pomeranz BA: Assessment of physiatrists' knowledge and perspectives on the use of opioids: Review of basic concepts for managing chronic pain. Am J Phys Med Rehabil 1999;78:408–415.

Grossi G, Soares JJ, Angesleva J, et al: Psychosocial correlates of long-term sick-leave among patients with musculoskeletal pain. Pain 1999;80:607–619.

Gureje O, Von Korff M, Simon GE, et al: Persistent pain and well-being: A World Health Organization study in primary care. JAMA 1998;280:147–151.

Hallberg LR, Carlsson SG: Anxiety and coping in patients with chronic work-related muscular pain and patients with fibromyalgia. Eur J Pain 1998;2:309–319.

Harter M, Reuter K, Weisser B, et al: A descriptive study of psychiatric disorders and psychosocial burden in rehabilitation patients with musculoskeletal diseases. Arch Phys Med Rehabil 2002;83: 461–468.

Hasenbring M, Hallner D, Klasen B: Psychological mechanisms in the transition from acute to chronic pain: Over- or underrated? Schmerz 2001;15:442–447.

Hasenbring M, Marienfeld G, Kuhlendahl D, et al: Risk factors of chronicity in lumbar disc patients. A prospective investigation of biologic, psychologic, and social predictors of therapy outcome. Spine 1994;19:2759–2765.

Hasselstrom J, Liu-Palmgren J, Rasjo-Wraak G: Prevalence of pain in general practice. Eur J Pain 2002; 6:375–385.

Haythornthwaite JA, Sieber WJ, Kerns RD: Depression and the chronic pain experience. Pain 1991;46: 177–184.

Hellstrom C, Jansson B, Carlsson SG: Subjective future as a mediating factor in the relation between pain, pain-related distress and depression. Eur J Pain 1999;3:221–233.

Hellstrom C, Jansson B, Carlsson SG: Perceived future in chronic pain: The relationship between outlook on future and empirically derived psychological patient profiles. Eur J Pain 2000;4:283–290.

Hildebrandt J, Pfingsten M, Saur P, et al: Prediction of success from a multidisciplinary treatment program for chronic low back pain. Spine 1997;22:990–1001.

Hiller W, Fichter MM, Rief W: A controlled treatment study of somatoform disorders including analysis of healthcare utilization and cost-effectiveness. J Psychosom Res 2003;54:369–380.

Hoffman NG, Olofsson O, Salen B, et al: Prevalence of abuse and dependency in chronic pain patients. Int J Addict 1995;30:919–927.

Hotopf M, Mayou R, Wadsworth M, et al: Temporal relationships between physical symptoms and psychiatric disorder. Results from a national birth cohort. Br J Psychiatry 1998;173:255–261.

Hunt SP, Mantyh PW: The molecular dynamics of pain control. Nat Rev Neurosci 2001;2:83–91.

Jensen MP, Nielson WR, Romano JM, et al: Further evaluation of the pain stages of change questionnaire: Is the transtheoretical model of change useful for patients with chronic pain? Pain 2000;86: 255–264.

Jensen MP, Turner JA, Romano JM, et al: Coping with chronic pain: A critical review of the literature. Pain 1991a;47:249–283.

Jensen MP, Turner JA, Romano JM: Correlates of improvement in multidisciplinary treatment of chronic pain. J Consult Clin Psychol 1994;62:172–179.

Jensen MP, Turner JA, Romano JM: Self-efficacy and outcome expectancies: Relationship to chronic pain coping strategies and adjustment. Pain 1991b;44:263–269.

Karlsten R, Gordh T: How do drugs relieve neurogenic pain? Drugs Aging 1997;11:398–412.

Katon W, Sullivan M: Depression and a chronic medical illness. J Clin Psychiatry 1990;150(suppl):3–11.

Katz PP, Yelin EH: Prevalence and correlates of depressive symptoms among persons with rheumatoid arthritis. J Rheumatol 1993;20:790–796.

Keefe FJ, Beaupre PM, Weiner DK, et al: Pain in older adults: A cognitive-behavioral perspecitive; in Ferrell BR, Ferrell BA (eds): Pain in the Elderly. Seattle, IASP Press, 1996, pp 11–19.

Keefe FJ, Caldwell DS, Williams DA, et al: Pain coping skills training in the management of osteoarthritic knee pain: A comparative study. Behav Ther 1990a;21:49–62.

Keefe FJ, Caldwell DS, Williams DA, et al: Pain coping skills training in the management of osteoarthritic knee pain. II. Follow-up results. Behav Ther 1990b;21:435–447.

Keefe FJ, Crisson JE, Maltbie A, et al: Illness behavior as a predictor of pain and overt behavior patterns in chronic low back pain patients. J Psychosom Res 1986;30:543–551.

Kerns RD, Haythornthwaite JA: Depression among chronic pain patients: Cognitive-behavioral analysis and effect on rehabilitation outcome. J Consult Clin Psychol 1988;56:870–876.

Kerns RD, Rosenberg R, Jamison RN, et al: Readiness to adopt a self-management approach to chronic pain: The Pain Stages of Change Questionnaire (POSCQ). Pain 1997;72:227–234.

Kirsh KL, Whitcomb LA, Donaghy K, Passik SD: Abuse and addiction issues in medically ill patients with pain: Attempts at clarification of terms and empirical study. Clin J Pain 2002;18:S52–S60.

Kouyanou K, Pither CE, Wessely S: Medication misuse, abuse and dependence in chronic pain patients. J Psychosom Res 1997;43:497–504.

Kroenke K, Swindle R: Cognitive-behavioral therapy for somatization and symptom syndromes: A critical review of controlled clinical trials. Psychother Psychosom 2000;69:205–215.

Lackner JM, Carosella AM: The relative influence of perceived pain control, anxiety, and functional self efficacy on spinal function among patients with chronic low back pain. Spine 1999;24:2254–2260.

Lazarus RA, Folkman S: Stress, Appraisal, and Coping. New York, Springer, 1984.

Leino P, Magni G: Depressive and distress symptoms as predictors of low back pain, neck-shoulder pain, and other musculoskeletal morbidity: A 10 year follow-up of metal industry employees. Pain 1993;53:89–94.

Lethem J, Slade PD, Troup JDG, et al: Outline of fear-avoidance model of exaggerated pain perceptions. Behav Res Ther 1983;21:401–408.

Li L, Moore D: Acceptance of disability and its correlates. J Soc Psychol 1998;138:13–25.

Lin EH, Katon W, Von Korff M, et al: Effect of improving depression care on pain and functional outcomes among older adults with arthritis: A randomized controlled trial. JAMA 2003;290:2428–2439.

Lipowski ZJ: Somatization and depression. Psychosomatics 1990;31:13–21.

Long DM, Filtzer DL, BenDebba M, et al: Clinical features of the failed-back syndrome. J Neurosurg 1988;69:61–71.

Magni G, Marchetti M, Moreschi C, et al: Chronic musculoskeletal pain and depressive symptoms in the National Health and Nutrition Examination. I. Epidemiologic follow-up study. Pain 1993;53: 163–168.

Magni G, Moreschi C, Rigatti-Luchini S, et al: Prospective study on the relationship between depressive symptoms and chronic musculoskeletal pain. Pain 1994;56:289–297.

Magni G, Rigatti-Luchini S, Fracca F, et al: Suicidality in chronic abdominal pain: An analysis of the Hispanic Health and Nutrition Examination Survey (HHANES). Pain 1998;76:137–144.

Magni G, Schifano F, DeLeo D: Pain as a symptom in elderly depressed patients. Relationship to diagnostic subgroups. Eur Arch Psychiatry Neurol Sci 1985;235:143–145.

Mannion AF, Junge A, Taimela S, et al: Active therapy for chronic low back pain. 3. Factors influencing self-rated disability and its change following therapy. Spine 2001;26:920–929.

Mannion AF, Muntener M, Taimela S, et al: A randomized clinical trial of three active therapies for chronic low back pain. Spine 1999;24:2435–2448.

Mantyselka P, Ahonen R, Viinamaki H, et al: Drug use by patients visiting primary care physicians due to nonacute musculoskeletal pain. Eur J Pharm Sci 2002;17:210–216.

Mantyselka PT, Turunen JH, Ahonen RS, et al: Chronic pain and poor self-rated health. JAMA 2003; 290:2435–2442.

Marhold C, Linton SJ, Melin L: Identification of obstacles for chronic pain patients to return to work: Evaluation of a questionnaire. J Occup Rehabil 2002;12:65–75.

Maruta T, Swanson DW, Finlayson RE: Drug abuse and dependency in patients with chronic pain. Mayo Clin Proc 1979;54:241–244.

McCracken LM: Learning to live with the pain: Acceptance of pain predicts adjustment in persons with chronic pain. Pain 1998;74:21–27.

McCracken LM, Spertus IL, Janek AS, et al: Behavioral dimensions of adjustment in persons with chronic pain: Pain-related anxiety and acceptance. Pain 1999;80:283–289.

McCracken LM, Turk DC: Behavioral and cognitive-behavioral treatment for chronic pain: Outcome, predictors of outcome, and treatment process. Spine 2002;27:2564–2573.

McHugh PR: William Osler and the new psychiatry. Ann Intern Med 1987;107:914–918.

McHugh PR: A structure for psychiatry at the century's turn – The view from Johns Hopkins. J R Soc Med 1992;85:483–487.

McHugh PR, Slavney PR: Methods of reasoning in psychopathology: Conflict and resolution. Compr Psychiatry 1982;23:197–215.

McHugh PR, Slavney PR: The Perspectives of Psychiatry, ed 2. Baltimore, The Johns Hopkins University Press, 1998.

Meldrum ML: A capsule history of pain management. JAMA 2003;290:2470–2475.

Merskey H, Lindblom U, Mumford JM, et al: Pain terms: A current list with definitions and notes on usage. Pain 1986(suppl 3):S215–S221.

Miotto K, Compton P, Ling W, et al: Diagnosing addictive disease in chronic pain patients. Psychosomatics 1996;37:223–235.

Morley S, Eccleston C, Williams A: Systematic review and meta-analysis of randomized controlled trials of cognitive behaviour therapy and behaviour therapy for chronic pain in adults, excluding headache. Pain 1999;80:1–13.

Nicholson B: Responsible prescribing of opioids for the management of chronic pain. Drugs 2003;63: 17–32.

Nickel R, Raspe HH: Chronic pain: Epidemiology and health care utilization. Nervenarzt 2001;72: 897–906.

Nielson WR, Weir R: Biopsychosocial approaches to the treatment of chronic pain. Clin J Pain 2001;17 (4 suppl):S114–S127.

Novy DM, Nelson DV, Berry LA, et al: What does the Beck Depression Inventory measure in chronic pain?: A reappraisal. Pain 1995;61:261–270.

Novy DM, Nelson DV, Hetzel RD, et al: Coping with chronic pain: Sources of intrinsic and contextual variability. J Behav Med 1998;21:19–34.

Ohayon MM, Schatzberg AF: Using chronic pain to predict depressive morbidity in the general population. Arch Gen Psychiatry 2003;60:39–47.

Okifuji A, Turk DC, Sherman JJ: Evaluation of the relationship between depression and fibromyalgia syndrome: Why aren't all patients depressed? J Rheumatol 2000;27:212–219.

Ospina M, Harstall C: Prevalence of Chronic Pain: An Overview. Edmonton, Alberta Heritage Foundation for Medical Research, Health Technology Assessment, 2002, report No 28.

Patten SB: Long-term medical conditions and major depression in a Canadian population study at waves 1 and 2. J Affect Disord 2001;63:35–41.

Picavet HS, Vlaeyen JW, Schouten JS: Pain catastrophizing and kinesiophobia: Predictors of chronic low back pain. Am J Epidemiol 2002;156:1028–1034.

Pincus T, Williams A: Models and measurements of depression in chronic pain. J Psychosom Res 1999;47:211–219.

Portenoy RK, Foley KM: Chronic use of opioid analgesics in non-malignant pain: Report of 38 cases. Pain 1986;25:171–186.

Porter J, Jick H: Addiction rare in patients treated with narcotics. N Engl J Med 1980;302:123.

Price DD: Psychological and neural mechanisms of the affective dimension of pain. Science 2000;288: 1769–1772.

Ready LB, Sarkis E, Turner JA: Self-reported vs. actual use of medications in chronic pain patients. Pain 1982;12:285–294.

Reich J, Tupin J, Abramowitz S: Psychiatric diagnosis in chronic pain patients. Am J Psychiatry 1983;140:1495–1498.

Reid MC, Engles-Horton LL, Weber MB, et al: Use of opioid medications for chronic noncancer pain syndromes in primary care. J Gen Intern Med 2002;17:238–240.

Reis S: Expectancy theory of fear, anxiety, and panic. Clin Psychol Rev 1991;11:141–153.

Revenson TA, Felton BT: Disability and coping as predictors of psychological adjustment to rheumatoid arthritis. J Consult Clin Psychol 1989;57:344–348.

Riley JL III, Robinson ME: Validity of MMPI-2 profiles in chronic back pain patients: Differences in path models of coping and somatization. Clin J Pain 1998;14:324–335.

Risdon A, Eccleston C, Crombez G, et al: How can we learn to live with pain? A Q-methodological analysis of the diverse understandings of acceptance of chronic pain. Soc Sci Med 2003;56:375–386.

Robinson RC, Gatchel RJ, Polatin P, et al: Screening for problematic prescription opioid use. Clin J Pain 2001;17:220–228.

Romano JM, Syrjala KL, Levy RL, et al: Overt pain behaviors: Relationship to patient functioning and treatment outcome. Behav Ther 1988;19:191–201.

Rudy TE, Kerns RD, Turk DC: Chronic pain and depression: Toward a cognitive-behavioral mediation model. Pain 1988;35:129–140.

Rudy TE, Lieber SJ, Boston JR, et al: Psychosocial predictors of physical performance in disabled individuals with chronic pain. Clin J Pain 2003;19:18–30.

Savage SR: Addiction in the treatment of pain: Significance, recognition and management. J Pain Symptom Manage 1993;8:265–278.

Savage SR: Assessment for addiction in pain-treatment settings. Clin J Pain 2002;18:S28–S38.

Savage SR, Joranson DE, Covington EC, et al: Definitions related to the medical use of opioids: Evolution towards universal agreement. J Pain Symptom Manage 2003;26:655–667.

Schult ML, Soderback I, Jacobs K: Multidimensional aspects of work capability. Work 2000;15:41–53.

Severeijns R, Vlaeyen JW, van den Hout MA, et al: Pain catastrophizing predicts pain intensity, disability, and psychological distress independent of the level of physical impairment. Clin J Pain 2001;17: 165–172.

Sheftell FD, Atlas SJ: Migraine and psychiatric comorbidity: From theory and hypotheses to clinical application. Headache 2002;42:934–944.

Simon GE, VonKorff M, Piccinelli M, et al: An international study of the relation between somatic symptoms and depression. N Engl J Med 1999;341:1329–1335.

Smith GR: The epidemiology and treatment of depression when it coexists with somatoform disorders, somatization, or pain. Gen Hosp Psychiatry 1992;14:265–272.

Stenager EN, Stenager E, Jensen K: Attempted suicide, depression and physical diseases: A one-year follow-up study. Psychother Psychosom 1994;61:65–73.

Stewart WF, Ricci JA, Chee E, et al: Lost productive time and cost due to common pain conditions in the US workforce. JAMA 2003;290:2443–2454.

Stroud MW, Thorn BE, Jensen MP, et al: The relation between pain beliefs, negative thoughts, and psychosocial functioning in chronic pain patients. Pain 2000;84:347–352.

Sullivan M: DSM-IV pain disorder: A case against the diagnosis. Int Rev Psychiatry 2000;12:91–98.

Sullivan M, Katon W: Somatization: The path between distress and somatic symptoms. Am Pain Soc J 1993;2:141–149.

Sullivan MJ, Thorn B, Haythornthwaite JA, et al: Theoretical perspectives on the relation between catastrophizing and pain. Clin J Pain 2001;17:52–64.

Suter PB: Employment and litigation: Improved by work, assisted by verdict. Pain 2002;100:249–257.

Tan G, Jensen MP, Robinson-Whelen S, et al: Coping with chronic pain: A comparison of two measures. Pain 2001;90:127–133.

Taub A: Opioid analgesics in the treatment of chronic intractable pain on non-neoplastic origin; in Kitahata LM (ed): Narcotic Analgesics in Anesthesiology. Baltimore, Williams & Wilkins, 1982, pp 199–208.

Turk DC, Matyas TA: Pain-related behaviors: Communication of pain. Am Pain Soc J 1992;1:109–111.

Turk DC, Meichenbaum D, Genest M: Pain and Behavioral Medicine: A Cognitive-Behavioral Perspective. New York, Guilford Press, 1983.

Turk DC, Okifuji A: What features affect physicians' decisions to prescribe opioids for chronic noncancer pain patients? Clin J Pain 1997;13:330–336.

Turner JA: Comparison of group progressive-relaxation training and cognitive-behavioral group therapy for chronic low back pain. J Consult Clin Psychol 1982a;50:757–765.

Turner JA: Psychological interventions for chronic pain: A critical review. II. Operant conditioning, hypnosis, and cognitive-behavioral therapy. Pain 1982b;12:23–46.

Turner JA, Chapman CR: Psychological interventions for chronic pain: A critical review. I. Relaxation training and biofeedback. Pain 1982;12:1–21.

Turner JA, Jensen MP, Romano JM: Do beliefs, coping, and catastrophizing independently predict functioning in patients with chronic pain? Pain 2000;85:115–125.

Turner JA, Jensen MP, Warms CA, et al: Catastrophizing is associated with pain intensity, psychological distress, and pain-related disability among individuals with chronic pain after spinal cord injury. Pain 2002;98:127–134.

Turner JA, Romano JM: Psychological and psychosocial techniques: Cognitive-behavioral therapy; in Bonica JJ (ed): The Management of Pain. Philadelphia, Lea & Febiger, 1990, pp 1711–1720.

Van Damme S, Crombez G, Bijttebier P, et al: A confirmatory factor analysis of the Pain Catastrophizing Scale: Invariant factor structure across clinical and non-clinical populations. Pain 2002;96:319–324.

Van den Hout JH, Vlaeyen JW, Heuts PH, et al: Secondary prevention of work-related disability in nonspecific low back pain: Does problem-solving therapy help? A randomized clinical trial. Clin J Pain 2003;19:87–96.

Vendrig AA: The Minnesota Multiphasic Personality Inventory and Chronic Pain: A conceptual analysis of a long-standing but complicated relationship. Clin Psychol Rev 2000;20:533–559.

Vendrig AA, Derksen JJ, de Mey HR: MMPI-2 Personality Psychopathology Five (PSY-5) and prediction of treatment outcome for patients with chronic back pain. J Pers Assess 2000;74:423–438.

Verbunt JA, Seelen HA, Vlaeyen JW, et al: Disuse and deconditioning in chronic low back pain: Concepts and hypotheses on contributing mechanisms. Eur J Pain 2003;7:9–21.

Verhaak PF, Kerssens JJ, Dekker J, et al: Prevalence of chronic benign pain disorder among adults: A review of the literature. Pain 1998;77:231–239.

Vlaeyen JW, de Jong J, Geilen M, et al: The treatment of fear of movement/(re)injury in chronic low back pain: Further evidence on the effectiveness of exposure in vivo. Clin J Pain 2002;18:251–261.

Vlaeyen JW, Linton SJ: Fear-avoidance and its consequences in chronic musculoskeletal pain: A state of the art. Pain 2000;85:317–332.

Von Knorring L, Perris C, Eisemann M, et al: Pain as a symptom in depressive disorders. I. Relationship to diagnostic subgroup and depressive symptomatology. Pain 1983;15:19–26.

Von Korff M, LeResche L, Dworkin SF: First onset of common pain symptoms: A prospective study of depression as a risk factor. Pain 1993;55:251–258.

Von Korff M, Ormel J, Katon W, et al: Disability and depression among high utilizers of health care: A longitudinal analysis. Arch Gen Psychiatry 1992;49:91–100.

Vowles KE, Gross RT: Work-related beliefs about injury and physical capability for work in individuals with chronic pain. Pain 2003;101:291–298.

Waddell G, Newton M, Henderson I, et al: A Fear-Avoidance Beliefs Questionnaire (FABQ) and the role of fear-avoidance beliefs in chronic low back pain and disability. Pain 1993;52:157–168.

Weaver M, Schnoll S: Abuse liability in opioid therapy for pain treatment in patients with an addiction history. Clin J Pain 2002;18:S61–S69.

Weickgenant AL, Slater MA, Patterson TL, et al: Coping activities in chronic low back pain: Relationship with depression. Pain 1993;53:95–103.

Weisberg JN: Personality and personality disorders in chronic pain. Curr Rev Pain 2000;4:60–70.

Weisberg JN, Vaillancourt PD: Personality factors and disorders in chronic pain. Semin Clin Neuropsychiatry 1999;4:155–166.

Williams AC de C, Richardson PH: What does the BDI measure in chronic pain? Pain 1993;55:259–266.

Williamson GM, Schulz R: Pain, activity restriction and symptoms of depression among community-residing elderly adults. J Gerontol 1992;47:367–372.

Wilson KG, Mikail SF, D'Eon JL, et al: Alternative diagnostic criteria for major depressive disorder in patients with chronic pain. Pain 2001;91:227–234.

Yap AU, Tan KB, Chua EK, et al: Depression and somatization in patients with temporomandibular disorders. J Prosthet Dent 2002;88:479–484.

Michael R. Clark, MD, MPH
Associate Professor and Director, Adolf Meyer Chronic Pain Treatment Programs
Department of Psychiatry and Behavioral Sciences, Johns Hopkins Medical Institutions
Osler 320, 600 North Wolfe Street, Baltimore, MD 21287–5371 (USA)
Tel. +1 410 955 2126, Fax +1 410 614 8760, E-Mail mrclark@jhmi.edu

Clark MR, Treisman GJ (eds): Pain and Depression. An Interdisciplinary Patient-Centered
Approach. Adv Psychosom Med. Basel, Karger, 2004, vol 25, pp 28–40

# The Psychological Behaviorism Theory of Pain and the Placebo: Its Principles and Results of Research Application

*Peter S. Staats[a], Hamid Hekmat[b], Arthur W. Staats[c]*

[a]Department of Anesthesiology and Critical Care Medicine, Johns Hopkins
University, Baltimore, Md., [b]University of Wisconsin, Stevens Point, Wisc., and
[c]University of Hawaii, Manoa, Hawaii, USA

## Abstract

The psychological behaviorism theory of pain unifies biological, behavioral, and
cognitive-behavioral theories of pain and facilitates development of a common vocabulary
for pain research across disciplines. Pain investigation proceeds in seven interacting realms:
basic biology, conditioned learning, language cognition, personality differences, pain behavior, the social environment, and emotions. Because pain is an emotional response, examining the bidirectional impact of emotion is pivotal to understanding pain. Emotion influences
each of the other areas of interest and causes the impact of each factor to amplify or diminish in an additive fashion. Research based on this theory of pain has revealed the ameliorat-
ing impact on pain of (1) improving mood by engaging in pleasant sexual fantasies, (2)
reducing anxiety, and (3) reducing anger through various techniques. Application of the
theory to therapy improved the results of treatment of osteoarthritic pain. The psychological
behaviorism theory of the placebo considers the placebo a stimulus conditioned to elicit a
positive emotional response. This response is most powerful if it is elicited by conditioned
language. Research based on this theory of the placebo that pain is ameliorated by a placebo
suggestion and augmented by a nocebo suggestion and that pain sensitivity and pain anxiety
increase susceptibility to a placebo.

## The Psychological Behaviorism Theory of Pain

In 1996, we published a theory of pain that, through its recognition of the
multifaceted nature of pain, provides a unifying framework that embraces the

previously existing biological, behavioral, and cognitive-behavioral theories of pain [1, 2] This unification facilitates development of a common language that will enhance our research efforts by making them pertinent across many disciplines. As opposed to theories that rely more exclusively upon operant or cognitive principles, our theory recognizes the importance of the biological underpinnings of pain and how they influence and are influenced by psychological and behavioral events. Because it also derives strength from psychological behaviorism, the only unified theory of human behavior [3–5], we named our theory 'the psychological behaviorism theory of pain'.

We were not the first to recognize that pain arises from the combined stimulus of various psychosocial, cognitive, environmental, biological, and emotional factors. Our theory, however, was the first to characterize the various aspects or realms of pain investigation as basic to advanced, to integrate the various realms of pain, and to derive the principles that offer theoretical support in a consistent and coherent manner. Thus, our theory not only unifies all the various realms of pain, it also leads to predictions about aspects of pain that were previously poorly understood (e.g., the placebo response or the quantitative manner in which negative affective states affect pain).

Our first task in constructing this theory was to identify and define the realms of pain investigation in a way that would maximize development of a common language that can be used to describe similar events despite the biological, behavioral, or cognitive focus of an investigator.

## Deriving Theoretical Principles from a Consideration of the Realms of Pain

We identified seven major realms of pain investigation: biology, learning, cognition, personality, pain behavior, the social environment, and emotions. Any unifying theory of pain, therefore, must not only take these individual realms and their various roles into account, it must also deal with how they interact and influence each other.

### Biology

We consider the biological level the most basic area of pain investigation. It is certainly the first consideration for a practitioner who must first attempt to locate a pain generator in order to determine if curing an underlying problem will eliminate the patient's pain behavior (or outward and visible expression of pain). In line with the International Association for the Study of Pain's definition of pain as an unpleasant *emotional* experience [6] and with biological findings that locate the center of pain processing in the limbic system – the center of emotional processing – the first principle of our theory is that the emotional center is where mediation takes place between a biological stimulus and a behavioral response to pain. This explains very neatly why the same pain generator can have a widely different effect in different individuals.

### Learning

Except in newborns, pain generators do not operate on blank slates – individuals rely on what they have learned to modulate (at an emotional level) their behavioral response to pain, which often includes an emotional response. The next basic level of investigation in our scheme, therefore, involves learning, and, for this, we draw upon what is known about classical and operant conditioning as well as on our understanding of the complexity of human behavior.

Classical conditioning, which occurs when a neutral stimulus is paired a sufficient number of times with a pleasant or unpleasant experience, works with pain. Children who have experienced painful injections, for example, may begin crying (a negative emotional response) at the mere sight of a needle and syringe. Pain can only become a conditioned pain response after its first experience.

Classical conditioning, therefore, is emotional. Instrumental or operant conditioning on the other hand dictates motor responses. When a reinforcer is paired with a stimulus, the individual's motor reaction will respond to the reinforcer as well as to the stimulus. Reinforcers can be negative or positive and can weaken or strengthen the motor reaction. Intense stimuli tend to invoke a conditioned response fairly quickly. Removal of a reinforcer from a motor response will eventually cause the conditioning to become extinct. Operant conditioning works like this in pain: if a person feels pain upon walking, and the pain is relieved by sitting, the person will choose sitting over walking. That is, the act of sitting will be reinforced by the withdrawal of the pain.

A consideration of pain teaches us that the behaviors an individual acquires through classical (emotional) and operant (motor) conditioning are intimately related because pain stimuli are reinforcers. First, a nociceptive stimulus elicits a negative emotional response that can be conditioned to any associated stimulus. Then, removal of a nociceptive stimulus can reinforce the behavior that preceded the removal. Pain behavior goes beyond these two reactions, however, because the same nociceptive stimulus that elicits a negative emotional response can itself directly elicit motor behavior (that will allow the individual to avoid the pain). We all approach the carrot and avoid the stick. Eliciting such an approach or avoidance is called directive stimuli.

### Cognition

Humans are not donkeys, however; our gift of language has made the basic tenets of conditioning influence our behavior in complicated ways. Conditioning pairs individual words with strong emotional responses (positive or negative) that operate as reinforcing and/or directing stimuli. In fact, individual cognitive characteristics (emotional states) differ according to how many emotional words the individual has learned and experienced. Combinations of words act in the same way to elicit positive or negative emotional responses of varying degrees. And these words have power whether we say, read, or hear them.

When we view this complex phenomenon from a perspective that seeks to account for the equally complex experience of pain, we realize that the continuing profusion of positive and negative emotional responses elicited by language combines to create an emotional state, which will be positive if the positive responses outweigh negative ones and negative if the opposite is true. An emotional state is like a porridge that is sweetened with honey and seasoned with salt. It not only has its own characteristic in response to the sum of the ingredients, it absorbs any further additions. Thus, at some point, additional experiences can tip the balance and change an individual's emotional state from positive to negative or vice versa. An emotional state can also change the positive/negative impact of an additional experience (adding more sugar intensifies sweetness). Emotional states may be experienced as short-lived or persistent moods.

This understanding of emotional states joined with that of pain as an unpleasant emotion allows us to see how a negative emotional state can intensify the experience of pain and vice versa. On the other hand, a positive emotional state can reduce the experience of pain and vice versa. Thus, patients suffering chronic pain often have comorbid depression, which, in turn, intensifies the pain. Depression arising from non-pain-related events can also have a deleterious effect on pain.

*Personality*

In order to explain the pain phenomenon, our theory must locate these biological/behavioral/learning/cognition principles firmly within a framework that also explains the impact of personality differences.

Our theory of personality, which arises from the basic behavioral principles we reviewed above, defines personality as the sum of three different learned repertoires of behavior. First, our personality is a creation of our extensive and complex repertoire of language-cognition responses. This repertoire contains subrepertoires that differ from individual to individual and acts (thinking, planning, communicating) that arise from these individualized subrepertoires. Second, our personality is shaped by the emotional responses we have learned to pair with various stimuli. Third, our personality includes our sensory-motor responses to conditioned stimuli, some of which are so complicated (making pottery) that they comprise repertoires themselves.

Thus, what we call 'personality' is the behavioral manifestation of our conditioning and our learning our basic behavioral repertoire. But biology also plays a role. Our theory holds that biological conditions (normal or abnormal) mediate the translation of learned experiences (past or present) into basic behavioral repertoires and that biological factors come into play again to influence our ability to sense (recognize) and respond to current lessons and to retain what we have learned. At any given time, an individual's behavior will affect the current environment, making changes that will affect future behavior in an ongoing interaction.

This theory of personality, thus, unifies what we know about the actions of biological and emotional variables with basic principles of learning and conditioning.

### Pain Behavior

Pain, of course, affects and is affected by personality repertoires. Beginning again with the language-cognition personality repertoire, it becomes clear that differences in emotional responses to words and phrases (language) play a large role in creating the differences we see in how individuals perceive and react to pain. In the case of pain arising from cancer, for example, a patient who associates 'cancer' with 'death' is likely to exhibit or report more suffering than a patient who associates 'cancer' with 'cure'. Expanding this relationship to the more complex language repertoire that oversees each individual's language labeling 'style' (pessimistic, optimistic), let us hypothesize that a pessimistic individual will exhibit or report more suffering than an optimistic individual from an equally painful condition. The second behavioral repertoire, an individual's set of learned emotional responses to various stimuli, obviously plays a role in determining if that person's emotional state is positive or negative, especially if the responses are accompanied by a series of reinforcers and directive stimuli. As noted above, the emotional state sets the stage for pain, either highlighting or diminishing its effect and how that effect is manifest. Finally, the sensory-motor repertoire will determine how an individual expresses pain behavior. A person given to flamboyant actions will likely exhibit more extreme pain behavior than a person whose sensory-motor repertoire comprises only reserved actions.

### The Social Environment

The social environment is a macrocosm in which all of the factors that are important for pain investigation on an individual level exert a similar bidirectional influence on pain on a cultural level. The biological level, for example, corresponds to those elements of the social environment that simply exist – the climate or geography – and which may or may not be altered by members of the society. The social environment oversees what we learn by controlling our stimuli. This, in turn, affects cognition and the development of the shared collective personality that we call culture. And this shared personality can exist in units as small as families or as large as factories. As an obvious example of the impact of the social environment, consider a person reared with a strong work ethic. That person is more likely than one reared without this cultural input to have a negative emotional reaction to disabling pain, which will, as we have shown above, enhance the experience of that pain.

*Emotion*
The bidirectional impact of emotion on pain can be seen at every level of pain investigation. And this impact affects not only the final sensation and expression of pain but also each of the major realms of pain. Thus, emotion influences and is influenced by biology, learning, cognition, personality, pain behavior, and the social environment, modifying and amplifying the experience of pain and the outcome of pain management. This influence occurs in an additive fashion – the addition of each factor increases the total impact. Thus, the emotional additivity principle predicts that a person's pain will increase if he or she experiences an additional negative emotion from another source. Likewise, pleasant experiences are expected to attenuate pain and relieve human suffering, and two positive emotional reactions will be more effective in attenuating pain than a positive and negative one.

An understanding of this bidirectional and additive role of emotion is pivotal to seeing the implications of the psychological behaviorism theory of pain.

## The Results of Research Supporting the Psychological Behaviorism Theory of Pain

*The Impact on Pain of Improving Mood by Engaging in Sexual Fantasies*
While trying to provide a general understanding of the psychological behaviorism theory to representatives of the national press, the first author said that positive thoughts ameliorate pain and that certain words and thoughts in certain circumstances would likely improve mood, e.g., the anticipation of having a meal when hungry or engaging in a sexual fantasy. The *National Inquirer* turned this remark into a headline to the effect that thinking about sex relieves pain. This prompted us to conduct a study in which we predicted that engaging in sexual fantasies alleviates acute pain, reduces anxiety and worry, and improves self-efficacy and that the impact of these fantasies would vary depending upon whether the participants rated them highly or moderately, with the best pain outcomes related to the highest-rated fantasies [7]. In this

randomized, controlled, cold pressor trial, we assigned 10 subjects each to a highly rated sexual fantasy, moderately rated sexual fantasy, nonsexual fantasy, or no-visualization control group. After obtaining baseline measures of pain, mood, worry, and self-efficacy, we asked the treatment groups to rehearse their fantasy and then visualize it during a second immersion in icy water. In support of our hypothesis, we found that visualization of only the highly rated sexual fantasies significantly alleviated pain, improved mood, reduced worry and tension, and enhanced self-efficacy.

### The Impact on Pain of Reducing Anxiety

The negative emotional conditions that accompany many types of pain manifest as anxiety, depression, and/or anger. Research exploring the effects of personality and mood states on pain supports the psychological behaviorism theory's tenet that such negative mood states influence the perception and response to pain [8].

The perceived ability to control anxiety is a personality variable because it is a permanent trait, and it can predict pain tolerance and endurance in individuals experiencing acute cold pressor pain [9]. Thus, individuals with low perceived control over anxiety tolerate less pain, show lower self-efficacy, display higher pain worry, and respond less favorably to relaxation and imaginal coping interventions. This means that anxiety management in clinical situations may attenuate the affective components of pain. In fact, an assessment of factors contributing to treatment outcome for chronic low back pain patients found a more profound positive effect associated with improving pain anxiety than with improving physical capacity [10].

Anxiety may be managed by behavioral interventions (relaxation, biofeedback, systematic desensitization, cognitive restructuring, and problem-solving) or by a variety of exposure and response prevention strategies aimed at teaching greater acceptance of fear, confronting anxiety directly, and preventing the patient from resorting to defensive avoidance maneuvers. The anxiety–pain link is further supported by the fact that antianxiety drugs, such as the benzodiazepine alprazolam, reduce pain ratings of noxious electric shock [11], and long-acting opioid analgesics reduce anxiety [12].

The Pain Anxiety Symptoms Scale (PASS) reliably measures the dimensions of anxiety that are sensitive to pain manipulation. The five factors identified as comprising pain-related anxiety are catastrophic thoughts, cognitive interference, coping strategies, physiological anxious arousal, and pain escape/avoidance. The degree of pain anxiety can significantly predict tolerance of acute pain [13] as well as a chronic pain patient's cognitive complaints [14], behavioral adjustment [15], physical complaints, and responsiveness to pain intervention [16, 17].

A study to determine how high and low perceived anxiety control interacts with the efficacy of pain-coping strategies split 60 participants into high or low anxiety control groups based on a median split in their scores on the Anxiety Control Questionnaire [18]. The members of each group were then randomized to receive either emotive relaxation (inducing relaxation by evoking positive affect) treatment, emotive relaxation treatment plus pain coping instructions, or no treatment (neutral instructions). Before and after the anxiety intervention, we measured anxiety, pain, and worry. Participants rehearsed their instructions before their second hand immersion.

As predicted, individuals with low anxiety control were significantly more susceptible to pain than those with high anxiety control and that the interventions had an independent and additive impact on pain threshold, pain tolerance, intensity, and perception. The coping intervention was more effective than the emotive treatment in attenuating pain of individuals with low anxiety control whereas those with high anxiety control responded favorably to both strategies.

Supporting the additivity principle of the psychological behaviorism theory, the combined effect of two positive coping strategies created a more potent positive emotional state than either component alone could have induced.

### The Impact on Pain of Reducing Anger

Because anger is a component of the experience of pain [19–21], suppressing anger and thereby increasing its intensity significantly predicts the experience of pain [22], lowers mood states and enhances pain [23]. To determine if managing anger through behavioral therapy facilitates pain coping, we conducted several experiments that examine the impact of various anger management techniques on pain.

#### Anger Flooding

In this study, we obtained baseline measures of cold pressor pain threshold, tolerance, and intensity as well as self-efficacy, pulse, worry, anxiety, anger, and mood and then randomly assigned the 60 subjects to one of three groups [24]. The anger flooding group subjects visualized a brief hierarchy of disturbing images of recent anger-evoking experiences and their associated self-verbalizations and then received treatment for both the imaginal and verbal components of the anger-evoking stressors. The neutral imagery control participants visualized two neutral scenes, and the control group refrained from visualization. Then we administered a second cold pressor task and took outcome measures. As we predicted, the anger flooding intervention significantly reduced anger, distress, pain anxiety, state anxiety, trait anxiety, and worry and significantly improved mood states as well as pain threshold, tolerance, and intensity.

Anger Desensitization

To explore the effects of anger desensitization on the experience of acute pain, we obtained baseline measures of cold pressor test pain, worry, anxiety, and anger and randomly assigned 60 participants to one of following interventions: anger desensitization (visualizing anger-evoking events while relaxing with pleasant imagery), neutral imagery control, or no-treatment control [25]. When we repeated the measures after the intervention and analyzed our data, we found that the anger desensitization treatment significantly alleviated anger, pain anxiety, state anxiety, trait anxiety, and worry and significantly improved mood states, pain threshold, and pain tolerance.

These results confirmed our prediction based on the psychological behaviorism theory that the emotional management of anger by desensitization would facilitate coping with acute pain. They also confirmed our specific prediction that the anger desensitization group would report significantly less pain than the control groups.

Emotional Relaxation for Anger Management

To explore the effects on the experience of acute pain of managing anger with relaxation techniques, we randomly assigned 60 participants to three groups: a semantic relaxation intervention (visualizing pleasant events and engaging in coping self-instructions), a neutral imagery control, or a no-treatment control [26]. Prior to and after treatment, we measured cold pressor pain, worry, anxiety, and anger. Analysis of the data revealed that anger management by relaxation significantly alleviated anger, pain anxiety, state anxiety, trait anxiety, and worry and significantly improved mood states, pain threshold, and pain tolerance. These results confirmed our prediction that anger management by relaxation tactics would have beneficial effects on coping with acute pain.

*Psychological Behaviorism Therapy Treatment of Osteoarthritic Pain*

Psychological behaviorism therapy (PBT) is an intervention that integrates strategies derived from the principles of the psychological behaviorism theory of pain. Wells, Hekmat, and Staats explored the efficacy of PBT (stress management training, mood-enhancing imagery, pain-coping self-instructions, and a relaxation exercise designed to alleviate pain) in the management of chronic osteoarthritis pain in the elderly. This study randomized 35 patients (mean age 70.11 years) with a medical diagnosis of osteoarthritis of the knee to one of three groups: (1) PBT, (2) a self-efficacy, enhancing self-management intervention (based on the Arthritis Foundation's Self-Management Program), or (3) control. Both treatment groups showed gains in all outcome measures (pain, self-efficacy, personal resourcefulness, analgesic use, and psychological symptoms) that were not attained by controls. Compared with the self-efficacy group, the PBT significantly alleviated arthritic pain, reduced the intake of analgesics, and improved psychological symptoms, such as depression. Both the PBT and the self-management interventions led to significant improvements in managing pain and distress compared with controls, and both treatment groups maintained these therapeutic improvements and differences at 2-month follow-up (unpubl. data).

## The Psychological Behaviorism Theory of the Placebo

The psychological behaviorism theory of pain allows us to construct a parallel theory of the placebo in which we may consider the placebo for pain a stimulus (treatment condition) that reduces pain in the absence of a change in the biological condition producing the pain [27]. This placebo/treatment has the 'power' to reduce pain because it is a conditioned stimulus for a positive emotional response. Thus, little white sugar pills administered as a 'treatment' to an unsuspecting subject can elicit a positive emotional response and relieve pain because, in the past, that subject has paired little white pills (e.g., aspirin) with pain relief. The pill, however, is not the placebo; the suggestion that the pill offers efficacious treatment is the placebo, and the pill or other device is merely a conditioned stimulus.

The placebo is even more potent if, in addition to eliciting a positive emotional response, it involves language that enhances the positive emotional responses. What a doctor says to a patient (or a patient says to him/herself), therefore, may improve the patient's mood and reduce the impact of pain. In fact, the action of a placebo usually involves complex cognitive (language) mechanisms, and an assessment of how language elicits emotional responses is necessary to achieve an understanding of the placebo response.

Conditioned stimuli also elicit negative emotional responses that can exacerbate pain. Such a negative conditioned stimulus is called a negative placebo or 'nocebo'. According to our theory, language stimuli that elicit a negative emotional state will exacerbate pain.

## The Results of Research Supporting the Psychological Behaviorism Theory of the Placebo

*The Placebo and Pain*
For our first study [28] of the effect of the placebo on pain, we divided subjects into three groups and submitted them to a cold pressor test accompanied by (1) a placebo suggestion designed to elicit a positive emotional response,

(2) a nocebo suggestion designed to elicit a negative emotional response, or (3) an emotionally neutral suggestion. As predicted, pain was ameliorated by the placebo, exacerbated by the nocebo, and unchanged by the neutral intervention.

*Pain Sensitivity and Responsiveness to Placebo Suggestions*

The personality construct 'pain sensitivity' predicts fear of pain and pain avoidance behavior. We conducted a study to test our theoretical predictions that pain-sensitive individuals will experience pain more intensely than those who are not pain sensitive and that subjects receiving a positive placebo instruction regarding anticipated pain will experience less pain than those given a negative placebo, while pain scores of those receiving a neutral placebo instruction will fall in the middle [29]. We divided 72 subjects into high and low pain-sensitive groups based on their results in the Pain Sensitivity Index test. Further randomization subdivided the groups into those receiving a positive, negative, and neutral placebo suggestion (total 6 groups). Participants rehearsed their placebo suggestions and focused on them during a second exposure to ice water. Both the positive and negative placebo suggestion interventions significantly altered pain threshold, tolerance, and endurance in the expected directions. Participants with high pain sensitivity experienced more pain than did those with low pain sensitivity.

*Pain Anxiety and Responsiveness to Placebo Suggestion*

To determine the impact of multiple emotional responses elicited by a variety of means, including a placebo/nocebo on acute pain, we performed a randomized experimental study that examined the effect of pain anxiety (measured with the validated PASS) on the experience (threshold and intensity) and expression (tolerance and pain worry) of acute pain and the possibility of influencing this effect with placebo/nocebo/neutral suggestions [30].

Our 72 volunteers completed baseline measures of pain anxiety, pain worry, and mood. We used the median split in the pain anxiety scores to divide the group according to anxiety level (high/low) and collected scores of pain behavior, experience, and intensity during their first ice water immersion. We then subdivided each group so that a subgroup from each anxiety level would receive an instruction designed to elicit a positive (placebo), negative (nocebo), or neutral response. We then repeated the pain worry test and gathered second immersion pain and mood scores.

As expected, the pain scores differed significantly according to the level of pain anxiety and assigned placebo intervention, with best-to-worse scores reported in the following order: the low pain anxiety/placebo, high anxiety/placebo, low anxiety/neutral, low anxiety/nocebo, high anxiety/neutral, and high anxiety/nocebo groups. The placebo/nocebo intervention had the greatest effect in the high pain anxiety group. Thus, this study provided the first proof that the impact of pain anxiety and a placebo/nocebo response can be demonstrated by changes in pain, worry, and mood.

## Conclusion

One of the most important tenets of the psychological behaviorism theory of pain is that the complexity of the pain phenomena must be acknowledged in order to deal with pain successfully. Thus, the psychological behaviorism theory has been systematically constructed to interrelate the various levels involved in the study of pain – ranging from the biological to the psychological and social, some of which have been covered in a more specialized manner by other theoretical approaches.

In its application, the psychological behaviorism theory of pain provides a comprehensive framework that can (1) serve as a basis for empirical research while also incorporating and unifying the findings of research based on more specialized theories of pain and (2) enhance the ability of clinicians to understand and treat complex pain behavior.

## References

1    Staats P, Hekmat H, Staats AW: Psychological behaviorism theory of pain: A basis for unity. Pain Forum 1996;5:194–207.
2    Staats P, Hekmat H, Staats AW: Advantages of a unified science and a unified theory of pain. Pain Forum 1996;5:215–219.
3    Staats AW: Psychological behaviorism and behaviorizing psychology. Behav Anal 1994;17:93–114.
4    Staats AW, Eifert GH: The paradigmatic behaviorism theory of emotion: Basis for unification. Clin Psychol Rev 1990;10:539–566.
5    Staats AW, Heiby E: Paradigmatic behaviorism's theory of depression: Unified, explanatory, and heuristic; in Reiss S, Bootzin RR (eds): Theoretical Issues in Behavior Therapy. New York, Academic Press, 1985, pp 279–330.
6    International Association for the Study of Pain: Pain terms: A list with definitions and notes on usage. Pain 1979;6:249–252.
7    Staats PS, Hekmat H, Staats AW: Do sexual fantasies alleviate pain? (abstract). American Pain Society, October 1999.
8    Gatchel RJ, Weisberg JN: Personality Characteristics of Patients with Pain. Washington, American Psychological Association, 2000.
9    Feldner MT, Hekmat H: Perceived control over anxiety-related events as a predictor of pain behaviors in a cold pressor task. J Behav Ther Exp Psychiatry 2001;32:191–202.
10   McCracken LM, Gross RT, Eccleston C: Multimethod assessment of treatment process in chronic low back pain: Comparison of reported pain-related anxiety with directly measured physical capacity. Behav Res Ther 2002;40:585–594.
11   Janssen SA, Arntz A: No interactive effects of naltrexone and benzodiazepines on pain during phobic fear. Behav Res Ther 1999;37/1:77–86.

12 Haythornthwaite JA, Menefee LA, Heinberg LJ, Clark MR: Pain coping strategies predict perceived control over pain. Pain 1998;77/1:33–39.

13 Bishop KL, Holm JE, Borowiak DM, Wilson BA: Perceptions of pain in women with headache: A laboratory investigation of the influence of pain-related anxiety and fear. Headache 2001;41: 494–499.

14 McCracken LM, Iverson GL: Predicting complaints of impaired cognitive functioning in patients with chronic pain. J Pain Symptom Manage 2001;21:392–396.

15 McCracken LM, Spertus IL, Janeck AS, Sinclair D, Wetzel FT: Behavioral dimensions of adjustment in persons with chronic pain: Pain-related anxiety and acceptance. Pain 1999;80:283–289.

16 McCracken LM, Gross RT: Does anxiety affect coping with chronic pain? Clin J Pain 1993;9/4: 253–259.

17 McCracken LM, Faber SD, Janek AS: Pain-related anxiety predicts non-specific physical complaints in persons with chronic pain. Behav Res Ther 1998;36:621–630.

18 Hekmat H, Staats PS, Feldner M: Does anxiety control facilitate pain coping? (abstract). American Association of Behavior Therapy, November 2001.

19 Hertel JB, Hekmat H: Coping with cold-pressor pain: Effects of mood and covert imaginal modeling. Psychol Rec 1994;44:207–220.

20 Fernandez E, Turk DC: The scope and significance of anger in the experience of chronic pain. Pain 1995;61:165–175.

21 Martin PR, Seneviratne HM: The effects of food deprivation and a stressor on head pain. Health Psychol 1997;16:310–318.

22 Kerns RD, Rosenberg R, Jacob MC: Anger expression and chronic pain. J Behav Med 1994;17: 57–67.

23 Burns JB, Johnson BJ, Mahoney N, Devine J: Anger management style, hostility, and spouse responses: Gender differences in predictors of adjustment among chronic pain patients. Pain 1996;64:445–453.

24 Hekmat H, Staats PS, Staats A: Does anger control predict acute pain? (abstract). American Pain Society, March 2002.

25 Hekmat H, Staats PS, Staats A: Does anger desensitization facilitate coping with acute pain? (abstract). American Pain Society, March 2003.

26 Hekmat H, Staats PS: Does anger management by relaxation facilitate coping with acute pain? (abstract). Association for Advancement of Behavior Therapy, November 1999.

27 Staats PS, Doleys D, Hekmat H, Staats AW: The powerful placebo: Friend or foe?; in Warfield C, Rice A, McGrath P, Justins D (eds): Clinical Pain Management: Chronic Pain. London, Arnold, 2002, pp 273–284.

28 Staats PS, Hekmat H, Staats AW: Suggestion/placebo effects on pain: Negative as well as positive. J Pain Symptom Manage 1998;15:235–243.

29 Staats PS, Hekmat H, Staats AW: Pain sensitivity and responsiveness to placebo suggestions (abstract). American Pain Society, November 1998.

30 Staats PS, Staats A, Hekmat H: The additive impact of anxiety and a placebo on pain. Pain Med 2001;2:267–279.

Peter S. Staats, MD
Department of Anesthesiology and Critical Care Medicine, Division of Pain Medicine
The Johns Hopkins University School of Medicine
550 North Broadway, Suite 301, Baltimore, MD 21205 (USA)
Tel. +1 410 955 1818, Fax +1 410 502 6730, E-Mail pstaats@jhmi.edu

Clark MR, Treisman GJ (eds): Pain and Depression. An Interdisciplinary Patient-Centered
Approach. Adv Psychosom Med. Basel, Karger, 2004, vol 25, pp 41–62

......................

# Function, Disability, and Psychological Well-Being

*Patricia Katz*

Department of Medicine, Division of Rheumatology and Institute for
Health Policy Studies, University of California, San Francisco,
San Francisco, Calif., USA

### Abstract

Disability research in arthritis, as in disability research in general, has focused on
functional limitations and activities of daily living/instrumental activities of daily living
(ADL/IADL) disability, and has thus ignored a great deal of daily life. Unfortunately, the
areas of life that have been ignored may be those that are most important to individuals, and
may also be the most sensitive to the first signs of developing disability. The ability to
perform valued life activities, the wide range of activities that individuals find meaningful or
pleasurable above and beyond activities that are necessary for survival or self-sufficiency,
has strong links to psychological well-being – in some cases, stronger links than functional
limitations and disability in basic activities of daily living. A broader assessment of disability
has great potential for interrupting the disablement and distress process, thereby improving
the quality of life of individuals with arthritis. Assessment of the effects of arthritis, pain, or
other chronic health conditions should expand beyond assessment of functional limitations
and disability in basic activities to include assessment of disability in advanced, valued
activities.

## Introduction

This manuscript presents a discussion of how function, in particular
performance of 'valued life activities' (VLAs), is associated with psychological
well-being. VLAs are the wide range of activities that individuals find meaningful or pleasurable, above and beyond activities that are necessary for
survival or self-sufficiency [1]. Although the research discussed has been done
primarily among individuals with rheumatoid arthritis (RA), the concepts and
relationships described are currently being studied among individuals with

other chronic health conditions, such as asthma, chronic obstructive pulmonary disease, and multiple sclerosis. Nonetheless, since the bulk of research has focused on individuals with RA, the examples within this manuscript will also focus on RA. This manuscript will (1) examine models of disability and where the concept of VLAs fits into existing models, (2) discuss findings on the impact of RA on the performance of VLAs, and (3) discuss the relationship between disability in VLAs and psychological status. The manuscript will close with a summary of clinical implications of this research and suggestions for future research.

## Background: Disability Theory

Two models of disability have driven the bulk of disability research. The first is the International Classification of Impairments, Disabilities, and Handicaps (ICIDH; now known as International Classification of Functioning, Disability, and Health, or ICF) model, developed by the World Health Organization [2, 3]. It originally specified four components: disease, impairment, disability, and handicap. Impairments were defined as losses or abnormalities of structure or function at the level of the organ as the result of disease (e.g., swollen or painful joints). Impairments may lead to disability, the restriction or inability to perform activities, measured at the level of the individual. Handicaps may result from disability or impairment, and reflect disadvantage and role limitation at the level of the individual in a social context [4–6]. Although useful in some situations, problems have been reported using the ICIDH model as a research model [5].

The second model, developed by Nagi [8], and later adapted by the Institute of Medicine, also has four components: active pathology, impairment, functional limitation, and disability [6, 7]. Impairment is defined similarly to the ICIDH definition. Functional limitations and disability, covered in the ICIDH model under the concept of disability, are treated as separate entities in the Nagi model. Functional limitations are defined as limitation in performance at the level of the person, and disability refers to limitation in performance of socially defined roles and tasks at the level of the individual in a social context. The Nagi model does not include a concept parallel to handicap in the ICIDH model.

Verbrugge and Jette [7] expanded on the Nagi model to develop a model of the disablement process that included factors that may affect the pathway from pathology to functional outcomes (see fig. 1). In their model, pathology refers to biochemical and physiological abnormalities, or disease, injury, or congenital/developmental conditions (e.g., diagnosis of RA). Impairments are defined as dysfunctions or significant abnormalities in specific body systems that can have consequences for physical, mental, or social functioning

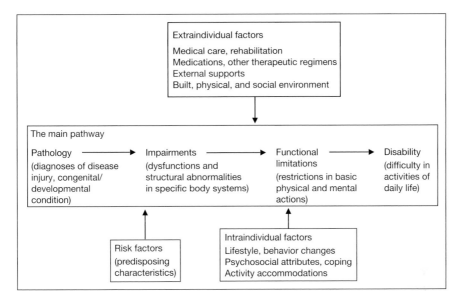

**Fig. 1.** Verbrugge and Jette model of disablement [adapted from 7].

(e.g., swollen or painful joints). Functional limitations refer to restrictions in performing generic, fundamental physical and mental *actions* used in daily life in many circumstances (e.g., walking, gripping). Finally, disability refers to difficulty performing *activities* of daily life (e.g., personal care, job, household management, recreation).

To illustrate the model, consider the case of RA. RA is a systemic condition that is characterized by joint pain and swelling, among other symptoms. Joint pain and swelling may lead to joint stiffness, limited joint range of motion, and weakness, which may lead to limitations in mobility, gripping, reaching, and other physical actions. Limitations in these actions may, in turn, cause difficulty in a wide range of activities from self-care to employment, to household maintenance, to hobbies.

Verbrugge and Jette [7] also recognized that certain predisposing factors could affect the presence or severity of impairments, functional limitations, or disability; these were termed 'risk factors'. For example, women with RA seem to experience greater pain and more functional limitations than men; persons with low education also seem to experience greater functional limitations. Sex and low education could thus be considered risk factors. In addition, certain factors can intervene in the process of disablement to reduce (or, in some cases, exacerbate) difficulties. These factors might include medical care, external supports such as assistance from others, psychosocial attributes such coping strategies, and activity accommodations such as modifying the way activities are performed. If disability is conceptualized as a gap between the capabilities of an individual and the demands of the environment, these interventions can lessen disability either by increasing capabilities or by reducing the demands of the environment.

When assessing disability, Verbrugge and colleagues [4, 7, 9] proposed that life activities be grouped into three categories: obligatory, committed, and discretionary activities. Obligatory activities are those required for survival and self-sufficiency, and include personal care, sleep and resting, walking, and local transportation. Committed activities are those associated with principal productive roles and household management, and include paid work, housework and food preparation, household repairs and yard maintenance, shopping and errands, and child and/or elder care. Discretionary activities are free-time pursuits, and include socializing with friends and relatives, entertainment away from home, hobbies and other leisure activities, active sports and physical recreation, and public service, religious, club, and adult education activities. The majority of disability research has focused on obligatory and, in some cases, committed, activities, and has ignored discretionary activities [4].

## What Is the Effect of RA on Function and Life Activities?

RA can produce significant functional limitations and disability. The functional impact of RA is commonly assessed with instruments such as the Health Assessment Questionnaire (HAQ) [10], which measures functional limitations in areas likely to be affected by arthritis, such as gripping, rising, mobility, and reaching, and disability in basic activities of daily living (ADLs) such as hygiene and eating. Studies also may assess some of the more complex tasks associated with independent community living called instrumental activities of daily living (IADLs; e.g., housework or transportation). The impact of RA may be clearly seen by focusing on functional limitations, ADLs, and IADLs. However, the same physical manifestations of RA that may cause difficulty in mobility or in performing a self-care activity may also cause difficulty in more complex leisure activities such as sewing or handwork, hobbies such as playing musical instruments, writing, or socializing with friends [11].

There has been much less research examining the impact of RA on this broader spectrum of life activities (committed and discretionary activities, in Verbrugge's terminology). The research that has been done has presented a consistent picture of impaired functioning in many domains of life activities. Yelin et al. [12] studied the impact of arthritis on a wide variety of life activities among individuals with RA and a group of controls with no arthritis. In every domain of function assessed, individuals with RA experienced significantly more activity losses over a 10-year period than did the controls. Work disability is a substantial problem for people with RA [13–17]. Individuals with RA report limitations in their ability to perform general household cleaning activities, laundry, shopping or errands, and cooking [18, 19] and they perform significantly less household work [20]. Nurturing activities associated with managing a household (e.g., making arrangements for others; taking care of sick people) and childcare are also affected by RA [18, 21]. Persons with RA have reported that RA interferes with performance of hobbies and pastimes and with sexual interest and activities [18, 22–27].

When RA affects function, individuals may experience difficulty with certain activities but be able to continue performing them, either with or without accommodations or modifications. However, individuals may also cease performing certain activities. These activities may cease because individuals become unable to perform certain actions, leading to the inability to perform specific activities, or individuals may relinquish less critical activities in order to have time and/or energy for others. Yelin et al. [12] noted that individuals with RA spent significantly more time in personal care activities (e.g., bathing, dressing, taking medicine) and sleep than controls. Kuper et al. [28] also noted that RA was associated with substantial time consumption, due mainly to extra time needed for ADLs, rest, and disease-related activities (e.g., physical therapy). Requiring more time for obligatory activities and for accommodating the additional time needed for rest and disease-related activities would, by default, leave less time for other types of activities. Which activities are maintained may depend on both the necessity of the activity for survival and self-sufficiency, and on the value the individual places on the activity.

### Adding the Concept of 'Personal Value' to the Assessment of Disability

Verbrugge [4] stated that the omission of a broader spectrum of activities in disability assessment reflects assumptions by researchers that the ADLs, IADLs, and employment are more important and that difficulty performing them was more significant. This assumption may not be true. The meaning, or 'value' attached to activities is person-specific, but may affect the impact of disability. In other words, some activities are more important or more meaningful to individuals than others. However, many of the activities identified as most important to persons with RA, and perhaps most closely tied to quality of life, are not measured in conventional functional assessments [4, 22]. Studies have shown that a large proportion of activities that are deemed important to individuals are outside the realm of ADLs, IADLs, and employment [5, 23, 24]. For example, Tugwell et al. [22] found that many activities identified as important by persons with RA were not included in conventional measurements. Conversely, many items on the conventional measures were not important to their patients. In two other studies, when persons with RA were asked what activities were affected by RA that most bothered them or what activities they most wanted to improve, only about half of the functions or activities mentioned were covered by the HAQ [23, 24]. The additional activities mentioned included a wide variety of leisure and recreational activities, childcare and other family roles, and work. Adding the concept of personal value to the assessment of disability is critical to determining the impact of functional problems on individuals' quality of life, but adds complexity to the assessment.

Katz [29] found that over a 5-year period, persons with RA lost over 10% of the activities that they had valued at the beginning of the period. Losses were seen in each of 13 domains of activity assessed, with the greatest losses in work-related (loss of 26.1% of activities valued at baseline), nurturing (19.1%), cultural and leisure (15.8%), public service/volunteer (15.5%), and social participation activities (13.8%). Compared to controls without RA matched for age, gender, and area of residence, persons with RA performed significantly fewer VLAs at the initial assessment (81.6% of the activities valued at baseline for the RA group, compared to 84.5% for controls; $p < 0.01$), and lost significantly more VLAs over the 5-year period (an average loss of 10.9% by persons with RA, compared to an average loss of 7.1% by persons without RA; $p < 0.01$). Half of the RA sample lost 10% of the activities they had valued at baseline, while only one third of the control group lost a similar proportion. At the end of the 5-year period, the difference between the RA group and the controls in the proportion of valued activities performed had widened – persons with RA were performing 70.7% of the activities they had valued at baseline while controls were performing 77.4%.

Another examination of the proportion of individuals with RA whose valued activities were affected by the disease is shown in table 1.[1] 'Affected' activities were those in which individuals reported either difficulty or that they were unable to perform because of their RA. It is readily apparent that individuals reported disability in all activity domains, although there is wide variability across domains in

---

[1]These data, as well as the data in the previous paragraph, are from the annual telephone interviews of the University of California, San Francisco Rheumatoid Arthritis (UCSF RA) panel. The previous paragraph's data are from interviews conducted from 1989 to 1993 (n = 512) [29]. The second set of data is from interviews conducted in 1998 and 1999 (n = 438). Panel retention rates averaged 93% from year to year. The panel was replenished with new members in 1995 and 1999. Detailed information on the UCSF RA panel is presented in references 29, 30, 46 and 47.

**Table 1.** VLA, disability prevalence and incidence

| VLA domains | % whose activities in domain were affected | % whose activities in domain were newly affected |
|---|---|---|
| Visiting with friends or family members in your home | 11 | 6 |
| Participating in religious activities or services | 28 | 11 |
| Leisure activities, such as going to movies, the theater, or restaurants | 30 | 10 |
| Going to social events, such as birthday parties, holiday parties, or family reunions, or visiting with friends or family members in their homes | 33 | 10 |
| Traveling or getting around your community by car or by public transportation | 36 | 14 |
| Taking care of family members, such as grandchildren, children, parents, or a sick spouse | 38 | 10 |
| Taking care of yourself, that is, activities such as bathing, washing, or getting dressed | 39 | 14 |
| Cooking, including food preparation | 39 | 8 |
| Walking, just to get around | 49 | 9 |
| Shopping or doing errands | 49 | 11 |
| Hobbies or crafts, such as sewing or woodworking | 57 | 15 |
| Working, that is paid employment | 68 | 11 |
| Other housework, such as vacuuming or dusting | 69 | 8 |
| Recreational activities, such as taking walks, gardening, or bicycling | 74 | 16 |
| Home maintenance, such as painting or heavy yard work | 85 | 5 |

Total n = 438; denominator for percentages is number who rated domain as important to them.

the prevalence of disability. Table 1 also presents the proportion of individuals whose activities were 'newly affected' in the second year of assessment, i.e., which were not affected in the first year but were affected in the second year, the equivalent of a 1-year incidence. The proportion of individuals with newly affected activities is much smaller, although considering that many of these individuals have had RA for over 20 years, the incidence of new disability is remarkable.

## What Is the Link between Function and Psychological Well-Being in RA?

Rates of depression and depressive symptoms[2] appear to be higher among individuals with RA than among the general population, with estimates ranging

[2]For the sake of simplicity, I will refer to both clinical diagnoses of depression and high levels of depressive symptoms suggestive of depression as 'depression'.

from 15 to 42% [30–33], depending on the sample and how depression was defined and assessed. For example, in a 3-year study, Katz and Yelin [30] found that 15–17% of subjects with RA were depressed in each of the 4 years studied, 5% were consistently depressed in every year, and over 29% were depressed in at least 1 year. The presence of depression in 1 year greatly increased the probability of depression in future years. For example, an individual who was depressed at the first assessment was over 6 times more likely to be depressed 2 and 3 years later, and was over 5 times more likely to be depressed 4 years later.

Among individuals with RA, many studies have demonstrated cross-sectional associations between depression and impaired functioning, primarily using measures of functional limitations or disability in ADL/IADL activities [30, 34–39]. For example, in the study just described, subjects who were depressed had poorer function as measured by the HAQ and were less likely to be working. Impaired functioning in a broader range of activities has also been correlated with depression, both in the general population [40–45] and in RA [46–48]. Among persons with RA, Katz and Yelin [46] noted that those who were depressed performed a significantly lower proportion of valued activities than did persons with RA who were not depressed.

These cross-sectional findings support an association between disability in life activities and depression, but do not answer the question of whether disability in life activities leads *to* depression. In a longitudinal study designed to address this question, subjects were assessed at three points in time [47]. Decline in function was measured as a substantial loss (10%) of valued activities or as a 0.5 increase in HAQ score[3] from time 1 to time 2; the onset of depression was assessed at time 3. (Individuals who were depressed prior to time 3 were excluded from analysis.) Loss of valued activities from time 1 to time 2 was strongly linked to the later development of new depression at time 3 [odds ratio (OR) 5.8, 95% confidence interval (CI) 2.0, 17.3]. In contrast, while a decline in basic function (increase in HAQ score) did predict the onset of depression when considered alone, it was not a significant risk factor when activity loss was also considered (OR 2.7, 95% CI 0.6, 12.3). The time lag between valued activity loss and development of depression made it clear that the loss of valued activities preceded, and was thus a risk factor for, development of depressive symptoms. Overall, these results suggest that the loss of VLAs, not simply functional impairment, is the aspect of functional decline that leads to the development of depressive symptoms.

[3]A change in HAQ score of 0.5 is equivalent to a 4-unit change, since scores increase/decrease in increments of 0.125. Scores range from 0 to 3.0, with higher scores representing worse function.

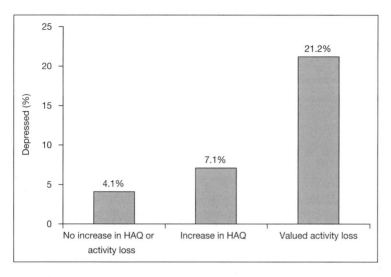

***Fig. 2.*** Effect of decline in basic function (i.e., increase in HAQ score) and valued activity loss on subsequent development of depression [from 47].

Interestingly, the overlap between loss of valued activities and decline in basic function was minimal. Forty-seven of the 319 women in the analysis experienced either loss of valued activities or decline in basic function. Only 6 (13%) experienced both. Fourteen experienced a decline in basic function and no loss of valued activities, and 27 had a loss of valued activities and no decline in basic function. Of the 33 individuals who lost 10% or more of the activities they had valued at time 1, 7 (21.2%) became depressed by time 3 (see fig. 2). Of the 14 individuals who had a decline in basic function without loss of activities, only 1 (7.1%) became depressed by time 3.

An additional longitudinal study confirmed the relationship between disability in valued activities and the later development of depression [49]. Again, individuals with RA were assessed at three time points. Individuals who experienced new disability in three or more activity domains from time 1 to time 2 were significantly more likely to develop subsequent depression at time 3 (fig. 3). After controlling for covariates, the odds of developing depressive symptoms were increased by 1.36 for every newly affected activity domain. In addition, new disability in recreational activities, social interactions, and the ability to get around one's community were specifically linked to the onset of new depressive symptoms (fig. 4). It appeared, then, that not only was the overall burden of valued activity disability linked to the development of depression, but that some activities were more important than others in the onset of depression.

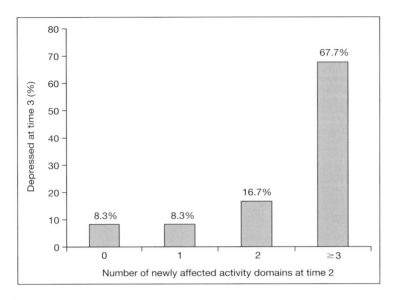

**Fig. 3.** Effect of disability in valued activity on subsequent development of depression. 67.7% of individuals who had 3 or more valued activities newly affected from time 1 to time 2 developed depressive symptoms between time 2 and time 3 [from 49].

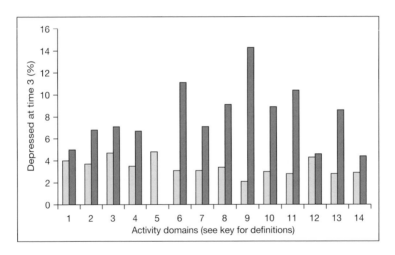

**Fig. 4.** Individuals who reported that specific activity domains (see key) were affected had higher rates of depression. Rates were significantly higher for social interaction, events outside home (6), recreation (9), and traveling, getting around community (11). 1 = Cooking; 2 = housework; 3 = home maintenance; 4 = shopping, errands; 5 = taking care of family members; 6 = social interaction events outside home; 7 = social interaction in home; 8 = entertainment; 9 = recreation; 10 = hobbies, crafts; 11 = traveling, getting around community; 12 = religious activities, services; 13 = writing, typing, other hand actions; 14 = working [from 49].

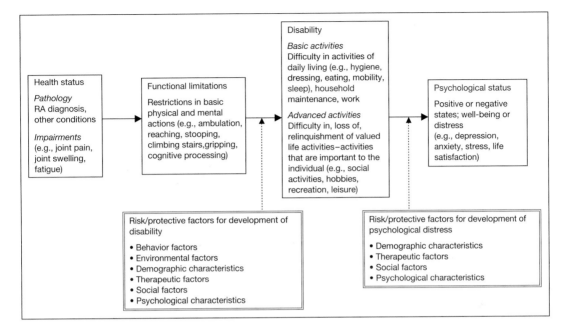

**Fig. 5.** Modification and extension of the Verbrugge and Jette model of disablement [7]. Modifications are: (1) combining impairment and functional limitations into a 'health status' category, (2) differentiation of types of disability (basic and advanced), and (3) suggestion that difficulty in basic activities will be associated with greater loss (relinquishment) of advanced activities. The model is extended to encompass the effects of disability on psychological well-being.

## What Are the Implications of the Relationship between Function and Psychological Well-Being for the Model of Disability?

Based on the findings just described, a modification and extension of the Verbrugge and Jette model of disablement [7] that encompasses the effects of disability on psychological well-being was developed (fig. 5). In this model, decrements in health status, which includes both pathology (e.g., presence of RA or other health conditions) and impairments (e.g., pain, joint deformities), lead to functional limitations (restrictions in basic physical or mental actions, such as walking, reaching, gripping, climbing stairs). These functional limitations, in turn, lead to disability. Disability is defined as difficulty in activities, inability to perform activities, or relinquishment of activities. Disability may be experienced in basic areas of function (roughly comparable to Verbrugge's categories of obligatory and committed activities) or in advanced activities (roughly comparable to Verbrugge's discretionary activities). Difficulty in basic activities is also likely to lead to relinquishment of advanced activities, due to increased time and energy requirements needed for basic activities. This aspect of the model has not yet been tested, however, although previous research suggesting a hierarchical development of disability supports the hypothesis [48, 50]. Although disability in basic activities may be associated with psychological distress, in general, research shows that it is disability in these more advanced activities that is associated with the onset of psychological distress [47, 49, 50].

Additional support for the pathways shown in this model can be found. For example, Devins et al. [51] found that 'illness intrusiveness', defined as perceptions of how much RA 'interferes with' 13 life domains (work, active recreation, passive recreation, financial situation, relationship with spouse, sex life, family relations, other social relations, self-expression/self-improvement, religious expression, community and civic involvement, health, and diet) was significantly associated with depressive symptoms. The relationship was stronger among younger individuals than among older. In a study of older adults, those who stopped driving, which could potentially reduce their access to paid and volunteer work, community services and businesses, friends, and religious activities, were at increased risk of worsening depressive symptoms [52]. Among a group of noncancer patients, activity restriction was found to mediate the relationship between pain and depression [43]. In other words, pain was initially correlated with depression, but when the effect of pain on activities was considered, the relationship between pain and depression was no longer evident; instead the effect of pain on depression was seen through its effects of restricting activities. These findings were replicated among cancer patients [44], and, as also noted by Devins et al. [51], activity restriction was more distressing to younger individuals than to older ones. The relationship was also demonstrated in longitudinal analyses: as pain increased over time, activity restriction also increased, which was, in turn, associated with increases in depression [44]. In a community-based sample of persons with disabilities, Turner and Noh [53] found that increases in ADL disability were associated with increases in depression. Similar results were noted by Smedstad et al. [39] using the HAQ. A recent population-based study examining correlates of major depressive disorder reported that as depressive symptom severity increased, the proportion of individuals reporting impairment in major life role function also increased [54]. On a more positive note, Herzog et al. [40] found that more frequent participation in productive (e.g., housework, shopping) and leisure activities was associated with less depression and better physical health.

Additional work has been done to explore other components of the proposed model and to identify modifiers and mediators of the relationships shown

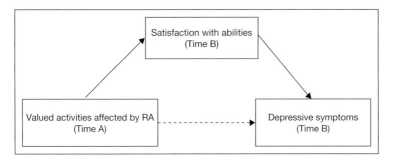

*Fig. 6.* Relationship between impact of RA on valued activities, satisfaction with abilities, and depressive symptoms. Satisfaction with abilities mediates the relationship between disability in valued activities and depression. When satisfaction was not accounted for, the impact of RA on valued activities at time A was a significant predictor of an increase in depressive symptoms at time B. When satisfaction was accounted for, it mediated the relationship between impact of RA and depressive symptoms, i.e., impact of RA was no longer a significant predictor of an increase in depressive symptoms. Valued activity impact predicted satisfaction, and satisfaction predicted depressive symptoms [56].

in the model. For example, performance of VLAs seems to be the type of functioning most closely linked to individuals' satisfaction with functional status [55]. Examining three measures of physical function – basic function (using the HAQ), a measure of functional limitations [the SF-36 Physical Component Score (PCS)], and the number of VLA domains affected by RA – all three measures were significantly correlated with satisfaction with function. However, while PCS accounted for 1% of the variation in satisfaction, and the HAQ accounted for less than 1%, performance of valued activities accounted for 9%. Satisfaction with abilities appears to mediate the relationship between loss of VLAs and depressive symptoms (fig. 6) [56]. Greater impact of RA on VLAs was found to be associated with greater dissatisfaction with abilities, which was then associated with higher depression scores. There was no direct relationship between VLA disability and depression when satisfaction with abilities was considered. Individuals who become disabled in valued activities and become dissatisfied with their level of functioning are more likely to become depressed; those who become disabled but do not become dissatisfied do not become depressed. The level of satisfaction with function may depend on the specific activities affected or on the value placed on those activities. These results underscore the need to consider individuals' interpretation of a functional loss or the value placed on the affected or lost activities and shed light on one way in which VLA disability might lead to depression.

## Clinical Implications of the Proposed Model

Existing evidence suggests that individuals with RA develop considerable disability in VLAs. Since RA is a chronic condition that often begins early in life and lasts for decades, VLA disability may develop and progress over many years. Performance of VLAs is the type of function most closely linked to satisfaction with functioning [55]. Loss of the ability to perform VLAs, particularly recreational activities and social interactions, has been shown to be a significant risk factor for the onset of depressive symptoms [43, 44, 47, 49]. Because of these established links, VLA disability appears to have the potential for considerable negative impact on individuals' psychological well-being and quality of life. Depression, in particular, has considerable economic and health costs. Economic costs attributable to depression, including direct medical, psychiatric, and pharmacologic care, mortality, and workplace absenteeism and reduced productive capacity, were estimated to be USD 43.7 billion in 1990 [57]. A more recent study estimated that depression produced an excess cost of USD 31 billion per year in lost productive work time alone [58]. Depressed persons have also been found to use more of other types of health services than nondepressed persons [30, 35, 59, 60], further increasing the economic costs. Depression has been shown to exert a negative influence on health in diverse ways, including inhibiting recovery following hip fracture surgery [61], increasing the risk of physical decline [62, 63], and increasing the risk for mortality [64, 65], and may lead to unwarranted changes in medications and overmedication due to the amplification of symptoms that depression may cause [66, 67]. Depression is also associated with poor treatment adherence, which may adversely affect treatment and health status [67]. Enabling individuals with RA to maintain VLAs or to maintain psychological well-being after VLA disability may avert some of the negative effects that appear to be associated with VLA disability.

Functional decline is an expected part of the disease process in RA. Medical treatment prescribed for RA, whether analgesic, disease-modifying antirheumatic drug (DMARD), or referral for surgery, is often prescribed in response to functional declines or to maintain function by alleviating pain, limiting damage, or replacing joints. In spite of these best efforts, functional impairments may continue to develop or worsen. Thus, it becomes clinically helpful to know that functional declines may create a risk for poor psychological outcomes for a patient. Awareness of worsening functional status can give the physician a cue to ask specific questions about function or activity losses. Answers to those questions may serve as cues for referrals for intervention.

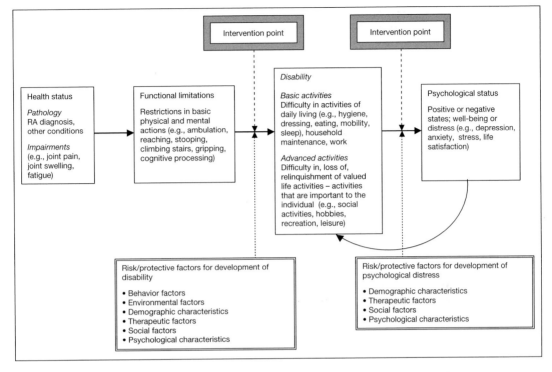

*Fig. 7.* Extension and modification of the Verbrugge and Jette model of disablement [7] showing points of intervention.

The theoretical model proposed offers two points of intervention (fig. 7).[4] The first intervention point is between functional limitations and disability, and would be intended to reduce disability. The individual may be able to make behavioral changes to lessen the impact of functional limitations in order to maintain activities (i.e., affect the pathway from functional limitations to disability). Such behavioral changes might include making modifications in the way activities are performed, replacing activities, or pacing oneself. The process of behavioral adaptation appears to be quite complex. Research by Gignac et al. [69, 70] shows that active efforts to minimize or circumvent disability through behavior accommodations are common, that the strategies used vary widely, and that individuals tend to vary adaptation strategies according to

[4]Medical therapies, such as medications or joint surgery, are not shown on the model. Escalante and Rincon [68] suggest that medical therapies can intervene at different stages in the disablement process in RA. Medications may affect pathology or impairment, joint surgery may reduce impairment and functional limitations.

the type of activity affected. Any intervention undertaken to increase behavioral adaptation would need to take such variation into account. Physical or occupational therapy or vocational rehabilitation may assist in this process.

Certain environmental and social factors may also affect the pathway from functional limitations to disability. For example, assistive devices are used relatively frequently and appear to be quite efficacious in reducing or resolving many functional limitations [71–73]. Having adequate help or personal assistance might also allow an individual to maintain activities. For example, having someone to drive her to a store, which has scooter-type shopping carts might enable an individual to continue to do her own shopping. Home, community, and workplace modifications may enable individuals with functional limitations to continue to perform activities; on the other hand, workplace or community characteristics may also create barriers to individuals with functional limitations, and hasten the transition from functional limitation to disability.

Therapeutic factors may lessen or delay the progress from functional limitation to disability. Through physical therapy, individuals may be able to maintain enough strength and range of motion in their joints to get around their community on their own. Finally, some individuals may have demographic or psychological characteristics that predispose them to the development of disability or to being able to maintain activities. For example, married individuals may be better able to enlist help than those who live alone [74], which would enable them to maintain valued activities. Individuals who are optimistic by nature or exhibit a greater degree of self-efficacy may also be better able to maintain activities [75, 76]. Conversely, individuals with low levels of education or who live alone may have few resources to draw upon to maintain activities [77].

The second intervention point is between disability and psychological status. These interventions would be intended to reduce the psychological impact of disability. Therapeutic interventions here might include counseling in addition to rehabilitation services. It may be important for individuals to have adequate emotional support to help them deal with their losses [78]. Adequate social support may also help individuals find replacements for lost activities, which has been linked to more positive affect [79]. A number of studies have shown that depression may lead to increases in disability or functional decline [62, 63, 80], creating a downward spiral in which disability leads to depression, and depression may then lead to further declines in psychological status (see fig. 7). This potential downward spiraling effect on physical and psychological well-being makes it all the more important to intervene in the disablement and distress process. In fact, in addition to being associated with psychological well-being, performance of valued activities has been linked to the maintenance of physical health by some researchers. Chipperfield and Greenslade [81] proposed that restriction of activities was stress-producing and equivalent to the stress produced by 'daily hassles', which has been found to have more profound negative health consequences than acute episodes of stress. Glass et al. [82] found that social (e.g., church, trips, playing cards, social groups) and productive (e.g., gardening, cooking, shopping, community work) activities that involve little or no enhancement of fitness lower the risk of mortality as much as fitness activities do.

These intervention points should be considered from a risk factor perspective as well. Knowing that individuals have characteristics that put them at risk of either becoming disabled or psychologically distressed can be a cue to provide preventive interventions. For example, women, who tend to experience more severe symptoms, individuals with low education, who may have few resources to draw on, and unmarried individuals who may be less able to enlist help in performing activities, may all be at increased risk of disability or psychological distress following disability.

## Suggestions for Future Research

One question that arises from the research described here is why disability in advanced activities is more closely linked to the development of depression than disability in more basic activities or functional limitations. It is possible that disability in discretionary activities, or VLAs, may be the first sign of disability that the individual perceives. This would suggest that there is a hierarchy in the development of disability, that disability may progress from more complex, advanced activities to basic activities (such as self-care) [50]. Some research suggests that individuals may relinquish complex activities in order to have time or energy to perform more basic activities necessary to maintain independence. In other words, the development of disability in discretionary activities may signal to the individual that worse things are to come. Once an individual has progressed to the point of needing help with ADL activities, their perspective may have changed and they may have come to terms with their disability.

A second major area of future research could focus on better identification of risk factors for progression from functional limitations to disability, and from disability to psychological distress. Identification of such risk factors would enable health care providers to target individuals who are at greatest risk. The third major area of future research would attempt to identify interventions that can interrupt the progression to disability and to psychological distress. These interventions might be behavioral, such as facilitating the identification and adoption of replacement activities. Duke et al. [79] found that individuals who were able to find replacement activities for activities that were lost as a result of illness had higher positive affect a year after illness onset. Social interventions might involve improving individuals' abilities to marshal emotional support from friends or family [83]. Interventions might also focus on psychological factors or cognitive strategies. Katz and Alfieri [84] found that perceptions of poor coping with RA were associated with greater dissatisfaction with function (which mediates the relationship between valued activity disability and depression). Unfavorable social comparisons regarding function (i.e., feeling that one had more difficulty with function than others of the same age) have also been linked to dissatisfaction with function [85]. Interventions to help individuals establish coping mechanisms that help them maintain a level of satisfaction with their changing abilities may also be effective in disrupting the path from disability to psychological distress.

## Conclusion

The ability to perform VLAs has strong links to psychological well-being – in some cases, stronger links than functional limitations and disability in basic ADLs. Identification of individuals who are at high risk for loss of valued activities due to health conditions, whether because of health status, behavioral factors, social resources, demographic characteristics, environmental factors, or other reasons, can perhaps create opportunities to avoid or lessen the development of disability. If activity loss does occur, interventions to moderate the impact of the loss may avoid negative psychological and quality of life outcomes.

Disability research in arthritis, as in disability research in general, has focused on functional limitations and ADL/IADL disability. In doing so, it has ignored a great deal of daily life, particularly advanced activities such as leisure, social, and recreational activities [4]. Unfortunately, the areas of life that have been ignored may be those that are most important to individuals with arthritis, and may also be the most sensitive to the first signs of developing disability. A broader assessment of disability has great potential for interrupting the disablement and distress process, thereby improving the quality of life of individuals with arthritis. Assessment of the effects of arthritis, pain, or other chronic health conditions thus should expand beyond assessment of functional limitations and disability in basic activities to include assessment of disability in advanced, valued activities.

## References

1   Ditto PH, Druley JA, Moore KA, Danks JH, Smucker WD: Fates worse than death: The role of valued life activities in health-state evaluations. Health Psychol 1996;15:332–343.

2	World Health Organization: International Classification of Impairments, Disabilities, and Handicaps. Geneva, WHO, 1980.

3	World Health Organizataion: International Classification of Impairments, Disabilities, and Handicaps. Short Version. Geneva, WHO, 2001.

4	Verbrugge LM: Disability. Rheum Dis Clin North Am 1990;16:741–761.

5	Johnston M, Pollard B: Consequences of disease: Testing the WHO International Classification of Impairments, Disabilities, and Handicaps (ICIDH) model. Soc Sci Med 2001;53:1261–1273.

6	Verbrugge LM: The iceberg of disability; in Stahl SM (ed): The Legacy of Longevity: Health and Health Care in Later Life. Newbury Park, Sage, 1990, pp 55–75.

7	Verbrugge LM, Jette AM: The disablement process. Soc Sci Med 1994;38:1–14.

8	Nagi SZ: Disability concepts revisited: Implications for prevention; in Pope A, Tarlow A (eds): Disability in America: Toward a National Agenda for Prevention. Washington, National Academy Press, 1991, pp 309–326.

9	Verbrugge LM, Gruber-Baldini AL, Fozard JL: Age differences and age changes in activities: Baltimore Longitudinal Study of Aging. J Gerontol B Psychol Sci Soc Sci 1996;51:S30–S41.

10	Fries J, Spitz P, Kraines R, Holman H: Measurement of patient outcomes in arthritis. Arthritis Rheum 1980;23:137–145.

11	Stewart A, Painter P: Issues in measuring physical functioning and disability in arthritis patients. Arthritis Care Res 1997;10:395–405.

12	Yelin E, Lubeck D, Holman H, Epstein W: The impact of rheumatoid arthritis and osteoarthritis: The activities of patients with rheumatoid arthritis and osteoarthritis compared to controls. J Rheumatol 1987;14:710–717.

13	Allaire S: Update on work disability in rheumatic diseases. Curr Opin Rheumatol 2001;13:93–98.

14	Barrett E, Scott D, Wiles N, Symmons D: The impact of rheumatoid arthritis on employment status in the early years of disease: A UK community-based study. Rheumatology 2000;39: 1403–1409.

15	Chorus A, Miedema H, Wevers C, van der Linden S: Labour force participation among patients with rheumatoid arthritis. Ann Rheum Dis 2000;59:549–554.

16	Wolfe F, Hawley DJ: The long-term outcomes of rheumatoid arthritis: Work disability: A prospective 18 year study of 823 patients. J Rheumatol 1998;25:2108–2117.

17	Yelin E: Musculoskeletal conditions and employment. Arthritis Care Res 1995;8:311–317.

18	Reisine S, Goodenow C, Grady K: The impact of rheumatoid arthritis on the homemaker. Soc Sci Med 1987;25:89–95.

19	van Jaarsveld CHM, Jacobs JWG, Schrijvers AJP, van Albada-Kuipers GA, Hofman DM, Bijlsma JWJ: Effects of rheumatoid arthritis on employment and social participation during the first years of disease in the Netherlands. Br J Rheumatol 1998;37:848–853.

20	Allaire S, Meenan R, Anderson J: The impact of rheumatoid arthritis on the household work performance of women. Arthritis Rheum 1991;34:669–678.

21	Ostensen M, Rugelsjoen A: Problem areas of the rheumatic mother. Am J Reprod Immunol 1992; 28:254–255.

22	Tugwell P, Bombardier C, Buchanan W, Goldsmith C, Grace E, Hanna B: The MACTAR Patient Preference Disability Questionnaire: An individualized functional priority approach for assessing improvement in physical disability in clinical trials in rheumatoid arthritis. J Rheumatol 1987;14: 446–451.

23	Verhoeven AC, Boers M, van der Linden S: Validity of the MACTAR Questionnaire as a functional index in a rheumatoid arthritis clinical trial. J Rheumatol 2000;27:2801–2809.

24	Hewlett S, Smith AP, Kirwan JR: Values for function in rheumatoid arthritis: Patients, professionals, and public. Ann Rheum Dis 2001;60:928–933.

25	Cornelissen P, Rasker J, Valkenburg H: The arthritis sufferer and the community: A comparison of arthritis sufferers in rural and urban areas. Ann Rheum Dis 1988;47:150–156.

26	Blake D, Maisiak R, Alarcon G, Holley H, Brown S: Sexual quality-of-life of patients with arthritis compared to arthritis-free controls. J Rheumatol 1987;14:570–576.

27	Albers JMC, Kuper HH, van Riel PLCM, Prevoo MLL, Van't Hof MA, van Gestel AM, Severens JL: Socio-economic consequences of rheumatoid arthritis in the first years of the disease. Rheumatology 1999;38:423–430.

28 Kuper IH, Prevoo MLL, van Leeuwen MA, van Riel PLCM, Lolkema WF, Postma DS, van Rijswijk MH: Disease associated time consumption in early rheumatoid arthritis. J Rheumatol 2000;27:1183–1189.

29 Katz PP: The impact of rheumatoid arthritis on life activities. Arthritis Care Res 1995;8:272–278.

30 Katz PP, Yelin EH: Prevalence and correlates of depressive symptoms among persons with rheumatoid arthritis. J Rheumatol 1993;20:790–796.

31 Frank RG, Beck NC, Parker JC, Kashani JH, Elliott TR, Haut AE, Smith E, Atwood C, Brownlee-Duffeck M, Kay DR: Depression in rheumatoid arthritis. J Rheumatol 1988;15:920–925.

32 Creed F, Ash G: Depression in rheumatoid arthritis: Aetiology and treatment. Int Rev Psychiatry 1992;4:23–34.

33 Abdel-Nasser AM, El-Azim SA, Taal E, El-Badawy SA, Rasker JJ, Valkenburg HA: Depression and depressive symptoms in rheumatoid arthritis patients: An analysis of their occurrence and determinants. Br J Rheumatol 1998;37:391–397.

34 Söderlin MK, Hakala M, Nieminen P: Anxiety and depression in a community-based rheumatoid arthritis population. Scand J Rheumatol 2000;29:177–183.

35 Hawley DJ, Wolfe F: Anxiety and depression in patients with rheumatoid arthritis: A prospective study of 400 patients. J Rheumatol 1988;15:932–941.

36 Peck JR, Smith TW, Ward JR, Milano R: Disability and depression in rheumatoid arthritis: A multi-trait, multi-method investigation. Arthritis Rheum 1989;32:1100–1106.

37 Fifield J, Reisine S, Sheehan TJ, McQuillan J: Gender, paid work, and symptoms of emotional distress in rheumatoid arthritis. Arthritis Rheum 1996;39:427–435.

38 Fitzpatrick R, Newman S, Archer R, Shipley M: Social support, disability and depression: A longitudinal study of rheumatoid arthritis. Soc Sci Med 1991;33:605–611.

39 Smedstad LM, Vaglum P, Moum T, Kvien TK: The relationship between psychological distress and traditional clinical variables: A 2 year prospective study of 216 patients with early rheumatoid arthritis. Br J Rheumatol 1997;36:1304–1311.

40 Herzog AR, Franks MM, Markus HR, Holmberg D: Activities and well-being in older age: Effects of self-concept and educational attainment. Psychol Aging 1998;13:179–185.

41 Lemon BW, Bengtson VL, Peterson JA: An exploration of the activity theory of aging: Activity types and life satisfaction among in-movers to a retirement community. J Gerontol 1972;27: 511–523.

42 Longino CF, Kart CS: Explicating activity theory: A formal replication. J Gerontol 1982;37: 713–722.

43 Williamson GM, Schulz R: Pain, activity restriction, and symptoms of depression among community-residing elderly adults. J Gerontol 1992;47:P367–P372.

44 Zimmer Z, Hickey T, Searle MS: Activity participation and well-being among older people with arthritis. Gerontologist 1995;35:463–471.

45 Williamson GM, Schultz R: Activity restriction mediates the association between pain and depressed affect: A study of younger and older cancer patients. Psychol Aging 1995;10:369–378.

46 Katz PP, Yelin EH: Life activities of persons with rheumatoid arthritis with and without depressive symptoms. Arthritis Care Res 1994;7:69–77.

47 Katz PP, Yelin EH: The development of depressive symptoms among women with rheumatoid arthritis: The role of function. Arthritis Rheum 1995;38:49–56.

48 Badley EM, Rothman LM, Wang PP: Modeling physical dependence in arthritis: The relative contribution of specific disabilities and environmental factors. Arthritis Care Res 1998;11: 335–345.

49 Katz PP, Yelin EH: Activity loss and the onset of depressive symptoms: Do some activities matter more than others? Arthritis Rheum 2001;44:1194–1202.

50 Williamson GM: Pain, functional disability, and depressed affect; in Williamson GM, Shaffer DR, Parmalee PA (eds): Physical Illness and Depression in Older Adults. New York, Kluwer Academic/Plenum Publishers, 2000, pp 51–64.

51 Devins GM, Edworthy SM, Guthrie NG, Martin L: Illness intrusiveness in rheumatoid arthritis: Differential impact on depressive symptoms over the adult lifespan. J Rheumatol 1992;19:709–715.

52 Fonda SJ, Wallace RB, Herzog AR: Changes in driving patterns and worsening depressive symptoms among older adults. J Gerontol B Psychol Sci Soc Sci 2001;56B:S343–S351.

53    Turner RJ, Noh S: Physical disability and depression: A longitudinal analysis. J Health Soc Behav 1988;29:23–37.

54    Kessler RC, Berglund P, Demler O, Jin R, Koretz D, Merikangas KR, Rush AJ, Walters EE, Wang PS: The epidemiology of major depressive disorder: Results from the National Comorbidity Survey Replication (NCS-R). JAMA 2003;289:3095–3105.

55    Katz PP, Yelin E, Lubeck DP, Buatti M, Wanhe LA: Satisfaction with function: What type of function do rheumatoid arthritis patients value most? Annual Meeting of the American College of Rheumatology, San Francisco, 2001.

56    Katz PP, Neugebauer A: Does satisfaction with abilities mediate the relationship between the impact of rheumatoid arthritis on valued activities and depressive symptoms? Arthritis Care Res 2001;45:263–269.

57    Greenberg PE, Stiglin LE, Finkelstein SN, Berndt ER: The economic burden of depression in 1990. J Clin Psychiatry 1993;54:405–418.

58    Stewart WF, Ricci JA, Chee E, Hahn SR, Morganstein D: Cost of lost productive work time among US workers with depression. JAMA 2003;289:3135–3144.

59    Katon W, Von Korff M, Lin E, Lipscomb P, Russo J, Wagner E, Polk E: Distressed high utilizers of medical care: DSM-III-R diagnoses and treatment needs. Gen Hosp Psychiatry 1990;12: 355–362.

60    Barsky AJ, Wyshak G, Klerman GL: Medical and psychiatric determinants of outpatient medical utilization. Med Care 1986;24:548–560.

61    Mutran EJ, Reitzes DC, Mossey J, Fernandez ME: Social support, depression, and recovery of walking ability following hip fracture surgery. J Gerontol B Psychol Sci Soc Sci 1995;50: S354–S361.

62    Bruce ML, Seeman TE, Merrill SS, Blazer DG: The impact of depressive symptomatology on physical decline: MacArthur studies of successful aging. Am J Public Health 1994;84: 1796–1799.

63    Penninx BWJH, Guralnik JM, Ferrucci L, Simonsick EM, Deeg DJH, Wallace RB: Depressive symptoms and physical decline in community-dwelling older persons. JAMA 1998;279:1720–1726.

64    Covinsky KE, Kahana E, Chin MH, Palmer RM, Fortinsky RH, Landefeld CS: Depressive symptoms and 3-year mortality in older hospitalized medical patients. Ann Intern Med 1999;130: 563–569.

65    Pulska T, Pahkala K, Laippala P, Kivela S: Follow-up study of longstanding depression as predictor of morality in elderly people living in the community. BMJ 1999;318:432–433.

66    DeVellis BM: Depression in rheumatological diseases. Baillières Clin Rheumatol 1993;7: 241–257.

67    Katon W, Sullivan MD: Depression and chronic medical illness. J Clin Psychiatry 1990;51(suppl): 3–14.

68    Escalante A, del Rincon I: The disablement process in rheumatoid arthritis. Arthritis Care Res 2002;47:333–342.

69    Gignac M, Cott C, Badley E: Adaptation to chronic illness and disability and its relationship to perceptions of independence and dependence. J Gerontol B Psychol Sci Soc Sci 2000;55: P362–P372.

70    Gignac MAM, Cott C, Badley EM: Adaptation to disability: Applying selective optimization with compensation to the behaviors of older adults with osteoarthritis. Psychol Aging 2002;17: 520–524.

71    Verbrugge LM, Rennert C, Madans JH: The great efficacy of personal and equipment assistance in reducing disability. Am J Public Health 1997;87:384–392.

72    Dellhag B, Bjelle A: A five-year follow-up of hand function and activities of daily living in rheumatoid arthritis patients. Arthritis Care Res 1999;12:33–41.

73    Nordenskiöld U, Grimby G, Dahlin-Ivanhoff S: Questionnaire to evaluate the effects of assistive devices and altered working methods in women with rheumatoid arthritis. Clin Rheumatol 1998; 17:6–16.

74    Penninx BWJH, van Tilburg T, Deeg DJH, Kriegsman DMW, Boeke AJP, van Eijk JTM: Direct and buffer effects of social support and personal coping resources in individuals with arthritis. Soc Sci Med 1997;44:393–402.

75  Persson LO, Berglund K, Sahlberg D: Psychological factors in chronic rheumatic diseases – A review. Scand J Rheumatol 1999;28:137–144.

76  Arnstein P, Caudill M, Mandle CL, Norris A, Beasley R: Self-efficacy as a mediator of the relationship between pain intensity, disability and depression in chronic pain patients. Pain 1999; 80:483–491.

77  Bosma H, van de Mheen D, Mackenbach JP: Social class in childhood and general health in adulthood: Questionnaire study of contribution of psychological attributes. BMJ 1999;318:18–22.

78  Neugebauer A, Katz PP: The impact of social support on valued activity, disability and depressive symptoms in RA. Arthritis Care Res, under review.

79  Duke J, Leventhal H, Brownlee S, Leventhal EA: Giving up and replacing activities in response to illness. J Gerontol B Psychol Sci Soc Sci 2002;57:P367–P376.

80  Kempen GIJM, Sullivan M, van Sonderen E, Ormel J: Performance-based and self-reported physical functioning in low-functioning older persons: Congruence of change and the impact of depressive symptoms. J Gerontol B Psychol Sci Soc Sci 1999;54:P380–P386.

81  Chipperfield JG, Greenslade L: Perceived control as a buffer in the use of health care services. J Gerontol B Psychol Sci Soc Sci 1999;54:P146–P154.

82  Glass TA, de Leon CM, Marottoli RA, Berkman LF: Population based study of social and productive activities as predictors of survival among elderly Americans. BMJ 1999;319:478–483.

83  Oxman TE, Hull JG: Social support and treatment response in older depressed primary care patients. J Gerontol B Psychol Sci Soc Sci 2001;56:P35–P45.

84  Katz PP, Alfieri W: Satisfaction with abilities and well-being: Development and validation of a questionnaire among persons with rheumatoid arthritis. Arthritis Care Res 1997;10:89–98.

85  Neugebauer A, Katz PP, Pasch LA: Effect of valued activity disability, social comparisons, and satisfaction with ability on depressive symptoms in rheumatoid arthritis. Health Psychol 2003;22: 253–262.

Patricia Katz, PhD,
University of California, San Francisco, Arthritis Research Group,
3333 California Street, Suite 270,
San Francisco, CA 94143–0920 (USA)
Tel. +1 415 476 5971, Fax +1 415 476 9030, E-Mail pkatz@itsa.ucsf.edu

Clark MR, Treisman GJ (eds): Pain and Depression. An Interdisciplinary Patient-Centered
Approach. Adv Psychosom Med. Basel, Karger, 2004, vol 25, pp 63–77

..........................

# Structural Models of Comorbidity among Common Mental Disorders: Connections to Chronic Pain

*Robert F. Krueger, Jennifer L. Tackett, Kristian E. Markon*

University of Minnesota – Twin Cities, Minneapolis, Minn., USA

## Abstract

Patterns of comorbidity among common mental disorders can be understood from the perspective of a model that regards mood, anxiety and somatization disorders as elements within an internalizing spectrum of disorder, and substance use and antisocial behavior disorders as elements within a separate externalizing spectrum of disorder. In this chapter, we evaluate the possibility of linking this model to literature on chronic pain. Evidence from psychosocial and biological perspectives points towards mechanisms that link chronic pain to internalizing disorders. Such evidence indicates that the internalizing-externalizing model may provide a useful framework for suggesting new directions for research on connections between chronic pain and mood, anxiety, and related disorders and traits.

Copyright © 2004 S. Karger AG, Basel

## Introduction

Common mental disorders – those involving mood dysregulation, anxiety, substance misuse, and antisocial behavior – are frequently comorbid [1–4]. Indeed comorbidity is often the rule, rather than the exception, in clinical practice [5, 6]. Nevertheless, patterns of comorbidity among common mental disorders are also systematic. Mental disorders involving depression and anxiety co-occur frequently enough that they can be conceptualized as elements within a broad spectrum of 'internalizing' disorders. In addition, mental disorders involving substance misuse and antisocial behavior can be conceptualized as elements within a broad spectrum of 'externalizing' disorders, a spectrum distinct from the internalizing spectrum. Together, the internalizing and externalizing spectra form a model of comorbidity among common mental disorders

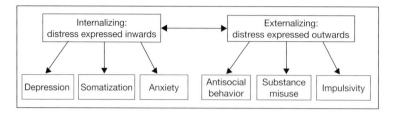

***Fig. 1.*** Heuristic diagram of the IE structural model of comorbidity among common psychopathological syndromes.

that has now been replicated by a number of independent research groups [7–12]. This kind of model is referred to as a structural model because it points towards the personality structures (the internalizing and externalizing spectra) that link various common mental disorders and help explain why common mental disorders show specific patterns of co-occurrence. Under this model, internalizing can be understood as a tendency to express distress inwards, placing the person at odds with themselves, and is manifested as syndromes that involve problems like depression, somatization, and anxiety. Similarly, externalizing can be understood as a tendency to express distress outwards, placing the person at odds with others and society, and is manifested in syndromes that involve problems like antisocial behavior, substance misuse, and impulsivity.

A heuristic guide to this model is presented in figure 1. As shown, syndromes involving depression, somatization, and anxiety are linked together as elements within the broader internalizing grouping. Similarly, syndromes involving antisocial behavior, substance misuse, and impulsivity are linked together as elements within the externalizing grouping. In addition, the internalizing and externalizing groupings are linked at a higher level by the presence of distress in all common mental disorders. That is, the model states that all common forms of psychopathology involve distress, which can be internalized or externalized, and subsequently expressed as the specific syndromes listed at the bottom of figure 1.

Emerging evidence suggests that this model organizes not only the observed, or phenotypic structure of common forms of psychopathology, but also underlying patterns of genetic risk for these syndromes [7]. That is, emerging evidence suggests that internalizing problems go together because they are linked by common genetic factors. Similarly, externalizing problems go together because they, too, are linked by common genetic factors – factors separate from those that link internalizing problems. The model therefore has high utility for organizing the search for genes that confer risk for the development of numerous common forms of psychopathology.

The goal of the current chapter is to extend this model to a new and relatively uncharted area at the interface between mental disorders and medical disorders: chronic pain. We begin with a review of literature pointing toward psychosocial and genetic mechanisms that may help to explain relationships between pain and other internalizing phenomena. We then turn to a discussion of some of our recent research locating somatic syndromes (including pain symptoms) within the internalizing spectrum of the internalizing-externalizing (IE) model. We conclude by discussing how the IE model could help organize research on psychosocial and genetic mechanisms that undergird the internalizing spectrum, including chronic pain.

## Psychotherapeutic Treatments for Depression and Chronic Pain

Cognitive behavioral therapy (CBT) techniques were originally developed in the 1950s and 1960s, initially to be used in treating depressive disorders [13]. However, the effectiveness of CBT techniques has also been demonstrated in individuals with chronic pain. Studies often show that CBT focused on pain-related symptomatology is effective in reducing both pain-related symptoms and depressive symptoms as evidenced by typical measures of these symptoms [14–16]. Benefits of CBT on pain-related symptoms have also been evidenced using an external criterion such as number of days of work missed following treatment [17]. These results have also been demonstrated in the use of CBT with children and adolescents [18]. In addition to CBT, behavioral techniques often used to treat depression and anxiety have been used as effective treatments for chronic pain [19]. Furthermore, even aerobic activity has been found to aid both depression and pain [20].

## Putative Mechanisms Underlying Psychotherapeutic Treatments

A related line of research has sought to identify common underlying mechanisms in depression and chronic pain that may explain why some treatments are effective for both. Some studies have identified similarities in cognitive processes between depressive and chronic pain individuals. For example, information-processing biases such as selective attention to negative stimuli, selective recall of mood congruent stimuli and interpretation of ambiguity as negative have all been related to both depression and chronic pain [21, 22]. Catastrophizing has also been related to increased levels of both depressive and pain-related symptoms [23–26].

Some common outcome variables have been investigated as they relate to effective treatment for both depression and chronic pain. In particular, changes in coping and self-efficacy seem to be an important measure of improvement in both depressive and pain-related symptoms following treatment [27, 28]. In this literature, coping is typically considered a cognitive variable related to the perceived use of effective strategies to deal with pain or depression symptoms. Problem-solving self-appraisal, or an individual's perception of their ability to problem-solve, has been identified as an important cognitive process involved in coping, and higher self-appraisal has been found to result in lower levels of pain and depression following treatment [29]. Similarly, perceived control has been linked with coping efficacy in both pain and depression [30, 31].

Romano and Turner [32, p. 30] provide a review of cognitive and behavioral frameworks that aim to explain the depression-pain association. They discuss an operant behavioral perspective (disorder results as a response to the environment), a more general behavioral perspective (pain becomes associated with displeasure in activities, activities are reduced to avoid pain, cycle of pain and depression results), and a cognitive perspective (disorder results from 'systematic negative distortions in cognitive processes'). Research exploring the applications of these perspectives in the realm of the pain–depression relationship, that is, targeting populations suffering from the comorbidity of chronic pain and depression, is lacking. Most of the emphasis on understanding applications of these theories has been in the depression literature [32], although the pain literature has become more active in this area recently.

*Summary*

Treatments such as the ones reviewed above have been shown to be effective in treating both chronic pain and depression and researchers have begun identifying similar underlying mechanisms that may explain the joint effectiveness of these treatments. However, most research to date that has included measures of both depression and chronic pain has investigated the effects of treatment for a particular population of chronic pain patients and measured changes in depression as well. It is less common for the selected sample to consist of patients with comorbid pain and depression, with the aim of understanding effectiveness of treatments for this comorbid condition, or extending the sampling scheme to patients with extensive and complex internalizing comorbidities (e.g., anxiety, depression, and pain). Thus, while some of the work in this area has begun to explore the common mechanisms underlying the effects of treatment for pain and depression, it is important for future research to test theories of treatment for complex patterns of internalizing comorbidity that are frequently seen in clinical settings.

## Psychopharmacological Treatments That Work for Depression and Chronic Pain

An influx of research over the last 15 years has provided compelling evidence that antidepressants can be used as an effective treatment for chronic pain. Tricyclics are a particular class of antidepressants that were hypothesized to be effective in treating pain. In support of this hypothesis, studies have generally found that tricyclics ameliorate pain symptoms [33, 34] and are effective in treating both pain and depressive symptoms [35]. Other antidepressants have also been studied in relation to pain, and some have been shown to have positive effects on pain symptoms [36–38] and on both pain and depressive symptoms [39, 40].

Hudson and Pope [41] reviewed the evidence on effectiveness of antidepressant treatments for a large class of disorders. Specifically, they identified major depressive disorder, bulimia, obsessive-compulsive disorder, panic disorder, attention deficit/hyperactivity disorder, cataplexy, migraine, and irritable bowel syndrome as a related class of disorders based on studies showing effective use of antidepressant treatments for them. Posttraumatic stress disorder and atypical facial pain nearly met the criteria to be classified in this grouping. Hudson and Pope termed this class of disorders that respond to antidepressants the 'affective spectrum disorder', based on the idea that response to treatment can be used to identify a similar pathophysiology among disorders. Hudson et al. [42] also recently presented a family study demonstrating significant coaggregation of major depressive disorder with other forms of affective spectrum disorder, expanded to also include dysthymic disorder, fibromyalgia, generalized anxiety disorder, posttraumatic stress disorder, premenstrual dysphoric disorder, and social phobia.

While most research in this area has looked at the impact of treatments for depression on symptoms of chronic pain, a recent study investigated the reverse relationship. Substance P, one of the best-understood neuropeptides, has been extensively studied in relation to pain. It has been widely established that substance P antagonists are helpful in alleviating pain [43]. Recently, evidence such as having similar patterns of distribution in the CNS, led one group of researchers to postulate that modulation of substance P may be linked to, or interact with, serotonin and norepinephrine pathways [44]. A randomized, double-blind, placebo-controlled study demonstrated efficacy in the treatment of depressive symptoms with a substance P antagonist, supporting the theory that substance P plays a role in regulating depression as well as pain [44].

## Putative Mechanisms Underlying Psychopharmacological Treatments

The documented high levels of comorbidity between depression and chronic pain have led some researchers to speculate that there is a common neurochemical association to account for the pain–depression relationship. Specifically, researchers have pointed to serotonin and norepinephrine to explain this connection [45]. It has been well-established in the literature that serotonin and norepinephrine play a role in depression [46, 47], and in the experience of pain [48]. In addition, endorphins in CNS have been shown to have a pain-modulating function and play a role in psychiatric disorders such as depression [32].

One model that has been proposed to explain the relationship between serotonin and norepinephrine in chronic pain and depression postulates that imbalances in serotonin and norepinephrine produce depression, while serotonin inhibits and norepinephrine enhances pain transmission [49]. According to this theory, an antidepressant in the tricyclic family would have the effects of alleviating both pain and depressive symptoms by acting on these neurotransmitters. Specifically, tricyclic antidepressants increase concentrations of both serotonin and norepinephrine [45], and most clinically effective antidepressants replicate this biochemical action [50]. Studies reviewed above regarding the use of antidepressants in treating pain, in particular the use of tricyclics, support the hypothesis. In addition, more recent work has sought to understand the relationship between substance P antagonists and depression. While still in its early stages, the connections between substance P receptors and serotonin and norepinephrine pathways have been a promising focus of study [51].

*Summary*

The use of antidepressants for chronic pain has received increasing attention through the last decade. In general, studies have shown antidepressants to be effective in treating chronic pain and in some studies, in treating both pain-related and depressive symptoms. The tricyclics have been the most widely studied, and differentiating types of antidepressants that are effective in treating pain may provide further information regarding the underlying neurochemical pathways. In addition, substance P is a neuropeptide associated with pain, and more recent work has found substance P antagonists to produce an antidepressant effect. Hypotheses of similar neurochemical pathways for pain and depression have primarily focused on the neurotransmitters serotonin and nor-epinephrine, which have been linked to both pain and depression. The use of pharmacological treatments for pain and depression is quickly growing in the literature, and future work in this area will provide important information in understanding the neurochemical similarities in depression and chronic pain.

## Quantitative Genetic Studies of Pain and Negative Emotions

Phenotypic studies are important as they demonstrate extensive relation-ships between pain and depressive phenomena. In themselves, however, they provide little information on why pain and depression are related to one another. Relationships between pain and depression may be mediated geneti-cally through genes acting on both; these relationships may also be mediated environmentally through common influences on both, or these relationships may be mediated through some combination of genetic and environmental influences. In order to properly disentangle different possible causal explana-tions, more complex biometric study designs are required.

Quantitative genetic studies of covariance differ in numerous ways, includ-ing the types of relatives examined (e.g., twins, sib pairs, extended families), the nature of the statistical models used (e.g., odds ratios vs. correlations), and the longitudinal nature of the design (e.g., cross-sectional vs. longitudinal). Ultimately, however, they are all based on the same premise: the strength of the relationship between two traits – where one trait is measured in one individual, and the other trait measured in a relative – should be proportional to the degree the relatives share genetic and environmental background. In a twin design, for example, this would be reflected in correlations between pain in one twin and depression in the other twin. To the extent these correlations are greater in monozygotic than dizygotic twins, genetic mediation of the relationship between pain and depression would be suggested.

Unfortunately, there have been few biometric studies of the relationship between pain and depression. Early family studies of chronic pain and depres-sion suggest that depression associated with chronic pain may partially reflect genetic vulnerability to depression. Relatives of individuals with both chronic back pain and depression, for example, have elevated levels of depression, but not alcoholism, relative to relatives of individuals with only chronic back pain [52, 53]. These findings suggest that the depression seen among individuals with chronic pain may sometimes reflect a general predisposition toward depressive phenomena, rather than sequelae of pain per se.

Recent studies of genetic and environmental relationships between pain and depression have tended to focus on specific forms of pain and traits associated with depression, such as anxiety and neuroticism. Reichborn-Kjennerud et al. [54], for example, recently investigated genetic and environmental relationships between back-neck pain and symptoms of depression and anxiety. The authors demonstrated that both pain and symptoms of depression and anxiety were heritable, the latter much more so. More importantly, approximately 60% of the correlation between pain and symptoms of depression and anxiety could be accounted for by genetic factors acting on both; the remaining correlation was attributed to environmental factors not shared between relatives. Overall, their results suggest that, to the extent back-neck pain and depression are correlated, the majority of that correlation is due to genetic factors acting on both; the remainder of the association is due to environmental factors largely specific to each individual.

Examination of other forms of pain, such as that associated with premenstrual symptoms, also supports the importance of genetic factors in relationships between depression and pain. Silberg et al. [55], for example, demonstrated that covariance between premenstrual symptoms and symptoms of anxiety, depression, and neuroticism can largely be attributed to genetic factors common to both sets of traits. Treloar et al. [56], similarly, reported a genetic correlation of 0.70 between premenstrual symptoms and lifetime major depression, and a genetic correlation of 0.62 between premenstrual symptoms and neuroticism.

### Molecular Genetic Studies of Pain and Negative Emotions

Evidence for genetic relationships between pain, depression, and other forms of negative emotion indicates that these phenomena share common molecular genetic substrates. Identifying these substrates – the particular genes and genetic systems involved in associations between pain and depression – is essential to understanding the etiology of both. Emerging evidence is revealing a number of neurogenetic systems involved in various forms of negative emotion, suggesting candidate substrates of internalizing phenomena.

Much of the existing knowledge about genes mediating the association between pain and depression has arisen from findings that systems known to be involved in pain are also involved in depression. The best examples of this, perhaps, are findings that the neuropeptide neurokinin (i.e., substance P, tachykinin) is involved in the etiology of depression. Numerous studies have established the role of neurokinin in nociception; emerging evidence suggests that it plays an important role in the experience of negative emotions such as anxiety and depression as well. Localization studies, for example, have demonstrated neurokinin activity in brain regions associated with regulation of negative emotion, such as the amygdala and dorsal raphe nucleus [44, 57, 58]. Also, as noted earlier, neurokinin antagonists show potent antidepressant effects in animals as well as in humans [44].

Various studies are beginning to elucidate the genetic mechanisms by which neurokinin regulates depression and other negative emotions. As a neuropeptide, neurokinin is directly encoded by the TAC1 gene, which in humans is located on the long arm of chromosome 7 in the 7q21-q22 region. TAC1 encodes a neurokinin precursor, preprotachykinin, that is spliced to form neurokinin. Neurokinin activity is also influenced by expression of the neurokinin receptor gene TACR1, which is located on the short arm of chromosome 2 in the 2p12 region.

Knockout studies in mice have demonstrated the role of TAC1 expression in depression and anxiety. Consistent with previous research on neurokinin and pain, TAC1 knockout mice demonstrate decreased nociception [59]. However, TAC1 knockout mice also express lower levels of depressive behavior than heterozygotes or wild-type mice. For example, TAC1 knockout mice evidence decreased immobility in behavioral despair paradigms such as forced-swimming and tail-suspension tests, and show decreased markers of depression in physiological paradigms [60]. TAC1 knockout mice express lower levels of anxiety in various paradigms as well. For example, TAC1 knockout mice are more active in the central area of an open field, spend more time in open maze compartments, show decreased latency to approaching food in a novel environment, and spend more time interacting socially with unfamiliar mice [60].

Knockout studies of the TACR1 gene have also demonstrated the role of neurokinin signaling in regulation of negative emotion. Mice lacking the neurokinin receptor gene show decreased levels of anxiety relative to heterozygotes and wild-type mice in a variety of paradigms. TACR1 knockout mice spend more time in open arms of an elevated plus maze, show decreased latency to approaching food in a novel environment, and, as pups, show decreased frequency of vocalizations when separated from their mother [58].

Overall, these studies demonstrate the role of neurokinin and neurokinin receptor gene expression in regulation of depression and anxiety. The mechanisms by which neurokinin and neurokinin receptor gene expression regulate negative emotion are not well understood, however. There is some indication that neurokinin systems interact with serotonergic pathways, but this is not established. For example, disruption of the TACR1 gene appears to increase firing of serotonergic neurons in the dorsal raphe nucleus [58], and is associated with desensitization of serotonin autoreceptors in a manner similar to that observed with sustained antidepressant use [61]. However, neurokinin antagonists apparently do not significantly influence serotonergic functioning [44], and there is some indication that TACR1 disruption influences serotonergic functioning indirectly through noradrenergic systems in the locus ceruleus [58].

In addition to neurokinin systems, other neurogenetic substrates are increasingly being implicated in the joint expression of pain and various forms of negative emotion. The opiate neuropeptides in particular represent another important class of neuromodulators involved in both pain and internalizing phenomena. Numerous molecular genetic studies suggest that various opiate neuropeptides are involved in pain and internalizing phenomena. Preproenkephalin gene knockout mice, for example, have altered nociceptive profiles and exhibit increased anxiety relative to wild-type mice [62]. Similarly, nociceptin knockout mice demonstrate elevated levels of anxiety in a variety of paradigms, as well as elevated pain thresholds [63].

Molecular genetic studies of pain and negative emotion in mice and other animals provide important information about the neuromolecular systems underlying internalizing phenomena. However, the role of these systems in regulating internalizing phenomena in humans remains poorly understood. As research on the behavioral genomics of negative emotion continues, it will become important to adopt a perspective that comprises a variety of phenomena simultaneously. Linkage and association studies focusing on pain, depression, and anxiety simultaneously, for example, will provide important information that would be missed if each were studied individually.

## The IE Model of the Structure of Common Mental Disorders: Recent Evidence of a Connection to Pain

As described earlier, the IE model is one evolving perspective that has the potential to encompass both pain and internalizing phenomena such as depression and anxiety simultaneously. This model originally emerged from our research on common mental disorders in general population samples, including unipolar mood, anxiety, substance use, and antisocial behavior disorders; chronic pain was not originally a focus of the model. However, we were recently able to study the model in the general health care setting [10]. Specifically, we evaluated the fit of the model to data from the World Health Organization (WHO) Collaborative Study of Psychological Problems in General Health Care [64], which was carried out in 15 study centers in 14 countries. Participating centers included Rio de Janeiro (Brazil), Santiago (Chile), Shanghai (China), Paris (France), Berlin and Mainz (Germany), Athens (Greece), Bangalore (India), Verona (Italy), Nagasaki (Japan), Groningen (The Netherlands), Ibadan (Nigeria), Ankara (Turkey), Manchester (UK), and Seattle, Wash. (USA). We were able to evaluate patterns of comorbidity among depression, somatization, hypochondriasis, neurasthenia, anxious worry, anxious arousal, and hazardous use of alcohol. The somatization symptom count included a number of pain-related symptoms (abdominal, back, joint, arms or legs, chest, headache, elsewhere), in addition to symptoms focused on gastrointestinal, cardiopulmonary, pseudoneurological, genitourinary, and skin complaints that were currently present and not medically explained.

In modeling the WHO data, we found that the best fitting model for the data from all the sites, modeled simultaneously, divided the syndromes into two distinct spectra or factors. The first factor (internalizing) was indicated by depression, somatization, hypochondriasis, neurasthenia, anxious worry, and anxious arousal. This factor was found to be separate from a factor indicated by hazardous use of alcohol. In addition, the strengths of the relationships between the underlying factors and their manifestations in specific syndromes (loadings) did not vary across countries.

These findings extend previous research on the IE model in a number of ways. The model fit data from diverse cultures, suggesting that the IE structure of these syndromes is relatively universal. In addition, the general health care setting and international focus of the research resulted in a different set of syndromes being modeled (somatization, hypochondriasis, and neurasthenia were not part of the model before this research was undertaken). Moreover, the inclusion of pain symptoms within the somatization symptom count suggests that medically unexplained current complaints of pain can be conceptualized as an element within the internalizing spectrum.

## Conclusions: The Internalizing Spectrum Conceptualization Can Inform Research on Chronic Pain

In this chapter, we have reviewed research on connections among internalizing syndromes (most often depression) and chronic pain. Research from various perspectives – psychosocial, psychopharmacological, quantitative-genetic, and molecular-genetic – points towards mechanisms that appear to link pain with internalizing syndromes. How can we understand and frame the evidence for these common mechanisms?

We suggest that the internalizing spectrum conceptualization could be a useful framework for understanding these connections and pointing towards directions for future research. As described earlier, the IE model has now been replicated by a number of independent research groups. Moreover, the internalizing spectrum component of the model bears a notable resemblance to the affective spectrum disorder concept, as well as to Tyrer's [65] concept of the general neurotic syndrome [66]. Thus, from a number of perspectives, the search for general mechanisms linking internalizing phenomena seems warranted, and the inclusion of chronic pain within the spectrum also seems warranted by our recent research in this area [10].

Some additional features of the IE model should also be emphasized in considering its ability to organize research linking internalizing disorders and chronic pain. Importantly, the model is dimensional and hierarchical in nature. What this means is that syndromes within the spectra are viewed as varying continuously both within and between persons, and are organized at continuously varying levels of connection among syndromes. These features of the model are described in more detail by Krueger and Piasecki [67], who also discuss statistical models that can be used to apply these features to empirical data. Thus, specific etiologic and pathophysiological factors can be conceptually and statistically linked to single syndromes, multiple syndromes, or the broad and overarching internalizing factor linking all syndromes within the spectrum. As a specific example, consider neurokinin. Research reviewed above suggests that this neuropeptide may play a very general role within the internalizing spectrum; the relevant genetic polymorphisms may be statistically linked to the overarching internalizing factor. Within the context of this more general genetic risk for internalizing problems, specific patterns of coping and cognitive styles could help to explain why the broad genetic risk for internalizing problems is expressed in specific persons as depression, anxiety, chronic pain, and so on, at specific times. We look forward to these kinds of empirical extensions of the ideas presented herein.

## References

1    Widiger TA, Sankis L: Adult psychopathology: Issues and controversies. Annu Rev Psychol 2000;
     51:377–404.
2    Kessler RC, McGonagle KA, Zhao S, Nelson CB, Hughes M, Eshleman S, Wittchen HU,
     Kendler KS: Lifetime and 12-month prevalence of DSM-III-R psychiatric disorders in the United
     States. Results from the National Comorbidity Survey. Arch Gen Psychiatry 1994;51:8–19.
3    Maser JD, Cloninger CR: Comorbidity of Mood and Anxiety Disorders. Washington, American
     Psychiatric Press, 1990.
4    Robins LN, Regier DA: Psychiatric Disorders in America. New York, Free Press, 1991.
5    Clark LA, Watson D, Reynolds S: Diagnosis and classification of psychopathology. Annu Rev
     Psychol 1995;46:121–153.
6    Widiger TA, Clark LA: Toward DSM-V and the classification of psychopathology. Psychol Bull
     2000;126:946–963.
7    Kendler KS, Prescott CA, Myers J, Neale MC: The structure of genetic and environmental risk
     factors for common psychiatric and substance use disorders in men and women. Arch Gen
     Psychiatry 2003;60:929–937.
8    Krueger RF: The structure of common mental disorders. Arch Gen Psychiatry 1999;56:921–926.
9    Krueger RF, Caspi A, Moffitt TE, Silva PA: The structure and stability of common mental
     disorders (DSM-III-R): A longitudinal-epidemiological study. J Abnorm Psychol 1998;107:
     216–227.

10   Krueger RF, Chentsova-Dutton Y, Markon K, Goldberg D, Ormel J: A cross cultural study of the structure of comorbidity among common psychopathological syndromes in the general health care setting. J Abnorm Psychol 2003;112:437–447.

11   Krueger RF, McGue M, Iacono WG: The higher-order structure of common DSM mental disorders: Internalization, externalization, and their connections to personality. Pers Indiv Diff 2001; 30:1245–1259.

12   Vollebergh WAM, Iedema J, Bijl RV, de Graff R, Smit F, Ormel J: The structure and stability of common mental disorders: The NEMESIS study. Arch Gen Psychiatry 2001;58:597–603.

13   Beck AT: Depression: Clinical, Experimental, and Theoretical Aspects. New York, Harper & Row, 1967.

14   Bradley LA, Young LD, Anderson KO, Turner RA, Agudelo CA, McDaniel LK, Pisko EJ, Semble EL, Morgan TM: Effects of psychological therapy on pain behavior of rheumatoid arthritis patients: Treatment outcome and six-month follow-up. Arthritis Rheum 1987;30:1105–1114.

15   Sharpe L, Sensky T, Timberlake N, Ryan B, Brewin CR, Allard S: A blind, randomized, controlled trial of cognitive-behavioural intervention for patients with recent onset rheumatoid arthritis: Preventing psychological and physical morbidity. Pain 2001;89:275–283.

16   Young LD: Psychological factors in rheumatoid arthritis. J Consult Clin Psychol 1992;60: 619–627.

17   Marhold C, Linton SJ, Melin L: A cognitive-behavioral return-to-work program: Effects on pain patients with a history of long-term versus short-term sick leave. Pain 2001;91:155–163.

18   Griffiths JD, Martin PR: Clinical- versus home-based treatment formats for children with chronic headache. Br J Health Psychol 1996;1:151–166.

19   Blanchard EB, Andrasik F, Evans DD, Neff DF, Appelbaum KA, Rodichok LD: Behavioral treatment of 250 chronic headache patients: A clinical replication series. Behav Ther 1985;16: 308–327.

20   Peters ML, Turner SM, Blanchard EB: The effects of aerobic exercise on chronic tension-type headache. Headache Q 1996;7:330–334.

21   Pincus T, Newman S: Recall bias, pain, depression and cost in back pain patients. Br J Clin Psychol 2001;40:143–156.

22   Turner JA, Jensen MP, Romano JM: Do beliefs, coping and catastrophizing independently predict functioning in patients with chronic pain? Pain 2000;85:115–125.

23   Hassett AL, Cone JD, Patella SJ, Sigal LH: The role of catastrophizing in the pain and depression of women with fibromyalgia syndrome. Arthritis Rheum 2000;43:2493–2500.

24   Haythornthwaite JA, Benrud-Larson LM: Psychological aspects of neuropathic pain. Clin J Pain 2000;16:S101–S105.

25   Hill A: The use of pain coping strategies by patients with phantom limb pain. Pain 1993;55: 347–353.

26   Roth RS, Geisser ME: Educational achievement and chronic pain disability: Mediating role of pain-related cognitions. Clin J Pain 2002;18:286–296.

27   Blanchard EB, Andrasik F: Psychological assessment and treatment of headache: Recent developments and emerging issues. J Consult Clin Psychol 1982;50:859–879.

28   Parker JC, Smarr KL, Buckelew SP, Stucky-Ropp RC, Hewett JE, Johnson JC, Wright GE, Irwin WS, Walker SE: Effects of stress management on clinical outcomes in rheumatoid arthritis. Arthritis Rheum 1995;38:1807–1818.

29   Witty TE, Heppner PP, Bernard CB, Thoreson RW: Problem-solving appraisal and psychological adjustment of persons with chronic low-back pain. J Clin Psychol Med Settings 2001;8:149–160.

30   Gibson SJ, Helme RD: Cognitive factors and the experience of pain and suffering in older persons. Pain 2000;85:375–383.

31   Jensen MP, Ehde DM, Hoffman AJ, Patterson DR, Czerniecki JM, Robinson LR: Cognitions, coping, and social environment predict adjustment to phantom limb pain. Pain 2002;95: 133–142.

32   Romano JM, Turner JA: Chronic pain and depression: Does the evidence support a relationship? Psychol Bull 1985;97:18–34.

33   Bryson HM, Wilde MI: Amitriptyline. A review of its pharmacological properties and therapeutic use in chronic pain states. Drugs Aging 1996;8:459–476.

34 Max MB: Antidepressant drugs as treatments for chronic pain: Efficacy and mechanisms; in Bromm B, Desmedt JE (eds): Advances in Pain Research and Therapy – Issue on Pain and the Brain: From Nociception to Cognition. New York, Raven, 1995.

35 Plesh O, Curtis D, Levine J, McCall WD: Amitriptyline treatment of chronic pain in patients with temporomandibular disorders. J Oral Rehabil 2000;27:834–841.

36 Jung AC, Staiger T, Sullivan M: The efficacy of selective serotonin reuptake inhibitors for the treatment of chronic pain. J Gen Intern Med 1997;12:384–389.

37 Onghena P, Van Houdenhove B: Antidepressant-induced analgesia in chronic non-malignant pain: A meta-analysis of 39 placebo-controlled studies. Pain 1992;49:205–219.

38 Sindrup SH, Gram LF, Brosen K, Eshoy O, Morgenson EF: The selective serotonin reuptake inhibitor paraxetine is effective in the treatment of diabetic neuropathy symptoms. Pain 1990;42:135–144.

39 Kudoh A, Ishihara H, Matsuki A: Effect of carbamazepine on pain scores of unipolar depressed patients with chronic pain: A trial of off-on-off-on design. Clin J Pain 1998;14:61–65.

40 Newburn G, Edwards R, Thomas H, Collier J, Fox K, Collins C, Cramer D, Reeves J: A comparison of the efficacy and tolerability of moclobemide given as a single dose or in three divided doses per day for the treatment of patients with a Major Depressive Episode (DSM-III-R). J Clin Psychopharmacol 1995;15/4S:10S–15S.

41 Hudson JI, Pope HGJ: Affective spectrum disorder: Does antidepressant response identify a family of disorders with a common pathophysiology? Am J Psychiatry 1990;147:552–564.

42 Hudson JI, Mangweth B, Pope HGJ, De Col C, Hausmann A, Gutweniger S, Laird NM, Biebl W, Tsuang MT: Family study of affective spectrum disorder. Arch Gen Psychiatry 2003;60:170–177.

43 Wahlestedt C: Reward for persistence in substance P research. Science 1998;281:1624–1625.

44 Kramer MS, Cutler N, Feighner J, Shrivastava R, Carman J, Sramek JJ, Reines SA, Liu G, Snavely D, Wyatt-Knowles E, Hale JJ, Mills SG, MacCoss M, Swain CJ, Harrison T, Hill RG, Hefti F, Scolnick EM, Cascieri MA, Chicchi GG, Sadowski S, Williams AR, Hewson L, Smith D, Carlson EJ, Hargreaves RJ, Rupniak NMJ: Distinct mechanism for antidepressant activity by blockade of central substance P receptors. Science 1998;281:1640–1645.

45 Fishbain DA, Cutler R, Rosomoff HL, Rosomoff RS: Chronic pain-associated depression: Antecedent or consequence of chronic pain? Clin J Pain 1997;13:116–137.

46 Blier P, de Montigny C: Current advances and trends in the treatment of depression. Trends Pharmacol Sci 1994;15:220–226.

47 Potter WZ, Manji HK: Catecholamines in depression: An update. Clin Chem 1994;40:279–287.

48 Hendler N: The anatomy and psychopharmacology of chronic pain. J Clin Psychiatry 1982;43:15–21.

49 Ward NG, Bloom VL, Dworkin S, Fawcett J, Narasimhachari N, Friedel RO: Psychobiological markers in coexisting pain and depression: Toward a unified theory. J Clin Psychiatry 1982;43:32–39.

50 Baker GB, Greenshaw AJ: Effects of long-term administration of antidepressants and neuroleptics on receptors in the central nervous system. Cell Mol Neurobiol 1989;9:1–44.

51 Rupniak NM: New insights into the antidepressant actions of substance P (NK1 receptor) antagonists. Can J Physiol Pharmacol 2002;80:489–494.

52 France RD, Krishnan KR, Trainor M: Chronic pain and depression. III. Family history study of depression and alcoholism in chronic low back pain patients. Pain 1986;24:185–190.

53 Krishnan KR, France RD, Houpt JL: Chronic low back pain and depression. Psychosomatics 1985;26:299–302.

54 Reichborn-Kjennerud T, Stoltenberg C, Tambs K, Roysamb E, Kringlen E, Torgersen S, Harris JR: Back-neck pain and symptoms of anxiety and depression: A population-based twin study. Psychol Med 2002;32:1009–1020.

55 Silberg JL, Martin NG, Heath AC: Genetic and environmental factors in primary dysmenorrhea and its relationship to anxiety, depression, and neuroticism. Behav Genet 1987;17:363–383.

56 Treloar SA, Heath AC, Martin NG: Genetic and environmental influences on premenstrual symptoms in an Australian twin sample. Psychol Med 2002;32:25–38.

57 Ribeiro-da-Silva A, Hokfelt T: Neuroanatomical localisation of substance P in the CNS and sensory neurons. Neuropeptides 2000;34:256–271.

58    Santarelli L, Gobbi G, Debs PC, Sibille EL, Blier P, Hen R, Heath MJS: Genetic and pharmaco-
      logical disruption of neurokinin 1 receptor function decreases anxiety-related behaviors and
      increases serotonergic function. Proc Natl Acad Sci USA 2001;98:1912–1917.
59    Zimmer A, Zimmer AM, Baffi J, Usdin T, Reynolds K, Konig M, Palkovits M, Mezey E:
      Hypoalgesia in mice with a targeted deletion of the tachykinin 1 gene. Proc Natl Acad Sci USA
      1998;95:2630–2635.
60    Bilkei-Gorzo A, Racz I, Michel K, Zimmer A: Diminished anxiety- and depression-related behav-
      iors in mice with selective deletion of the Tac1 gene. J Neurosci 2002;22:10046–10052.
61    Froger N, Gardier AM, Moratalla R, Alberti I, Lena I, Boni C, De Felipe C, Rupniak NMJ, Hunt SP,
      Jacquot C, Hamon M, Lanfumey L: 5-Hydroxytryptamine (5-HT)1A autoreceptor adaptive changes
      in substance P (neurokinin 1) receptor knock-out mice mimic antidepressant-induced desensitiza-
      tion. J Neurosci 2001;21:8188–8197.
62    Konig M, Zimmer AM, Steiner H, Holmes PV, Crawley JN, Brownstein MJ, Zimmer A: Pain
      responses, anxiety and aggression in mice deficient in pre-proenkephalin. Nature 1996;383:
      535–538.
63    Koster A, Montkowski A, Schulz S, Stube EM, Knaudt K, Jenck F, Moreau JL, Nothacker HP,
      Civelli O, Reinscheid RK: Targeted disruption of the orphanin FQ/nociceptin gene increases stress
      susceptibility and impairs stress adaptation in mice. Proc Natl Acad Sci USA 1999;96:
      10444–10449.
64    Ustun TB, Sartorius N: Mental Illness in General Health Care: An International Study. New York,
      Wiley, 1995.
65    Tyrer P: Neurosis divisible? Lancet 1985;i:685–688.
66    Andrews G, Stewart G, Morris-Yates A, Hold P, Henderson S: Evidence for a general neurotic syn-
      drome. Br J Psychiatry 1990;157:6–12.
67    Krueger RF, Piasecki TM: Toward a dimensional and psychometrically-informed approach to
      conceptualizing psychopathology. Behav Res Ther 2002;40:485–499.

Robert F. Krueger, PhD
Department of Psychology
N414 Elliott Hall, 75 E River Rd
Minneapolis, MN 55455 (USA)
Tel. +1 612 624 8204, Fax +1 612 626 2079, E-Mail krueg038@umn.edu

Clark MR, Treisman GJ (eds): Pain and Depression. An Interdisciplinary Patient-Centered
Approach. Adv Psychosom Med. Basel, Karger, 2004, vol 25, pp 78–88

..........................

# Neurobiology of Pain

*Michael R. Clark*[a], *Glenn J. Treisman*[b]

[a]Chronic Pain Treatment Programs and [b]AIDS Psychiatry Services,
Department of Psychiatry and Behavioral Sciences, Johns Hopkins Medical
Institutions, Baltimore, Md., USA

## Abstract

The neurobiology of pain has had extensive research directed at identifying the mechanisms of nociceptive transmission and integration. Clinical conditions of chronic pain
including phantom limb pain cannot be explained without an understanding of the complex
mechanisms of pain regulation. An overview of the neurobiological organization of the nociceptive system, from different pain fiber types to subcortical and cortical experiential centers, is presented, along with a brief description of the known cross talk within the system
and between pain pathways and those for other information. Finally, interactions between
affective, executive, and cognitive processes and pain experiences are described briefly.

## Introduction

The overly simple idea that pain is the central recognition of stimulation of
nociceptive receptors at the periphery of the nervous system has begun to give
way to the reality of the remarkable complexity of pain signals and integration.
It is clear now that nociceptive messages are integrated at every level of the
nervous system. Neurons that sense other stimuli can be recruited and report
pain sensations; silent neurons become active, and absent neurons (as in phantom pain syndromes) are read by the nervous system as active. It is also clear
that pain fibers talk to each other at peripheral fields, peripheral ganglia, the
spinal cord inputs, and at every higher level of integration. Chronic pain treatment will only become fully effective with the improved understanding of the
interrelationship between different pain mechanisms, and different levels of
pain integration.

The neurobiology of pain is described in numerous textbooks, chapters, and review articles [Bennett, 2000; Besson, 1999; Bolay and Moskowitz, 2002; Borsook, 1997; Cesaro and Ollat, 1997; Dickenson et al., 2002; Hunt and Mantyh, 2001; Price, 2000; Riedel and Neeck, 2001; Wall and Melzack, 1994; Zimmermann, 2001]. Complex interactions take place between structures of the peripheral and central nervous systems with modulatory mechanisms such as N-methyl-*D*-aspartate (NMDA) and opioid receptors within each component ultimately resulting in sensitization and desensitization of the system [Bennett, 2000; Bolay and Moskowitz, 2002; Riedel and Neeck, 2001]. Ongoing inflammatory/nociceptive or nerve injury/neuropathic stimulation cause sensory neurons to become electrically hyperexcitable and generate ectopic impulses manifested as spontaneous firing and abnormal responsiveness in neuroma endbulbs, regenerating sprouts, the dorsal root ganglia, areas of demyelination, and local uninjured axons. Afterdischarge and cross-excitation further distort and amplify nociception. Pathophysiological mechanisms range from remodeling of voltage-sensitive ion channels, upregulation of transducer molecules, and increased receptors in the cell membrane. Ectopic activity is a direct afferent signal but also produces central sensitization.

Not only is there cross talk between elements of the pain system, there is also cross modulation by systems that are not directly associated with pain. Emotional state, learning, exposure, and association all are impacted on by pain sensation, and appear able to modify sensory systems. Changes in peripheral nerves, spinal cord structures, and supraspinal structures contribute to sensory/discriminative abnormalities such as hyperalgesia and allodynia as well as affective/limbic pathophysiology such as depression and suffering [Hunt and Mantyh, 2001; Siddal and Cousins, 1995, 1998]. These alterations have been studied extensively in a variety of animal models and begin with the effects of local nerve injury. Changes proceed throughout the neuraxis including prolonged noxious stimulation and persistent abnormal ectopic neuronal inputs. Specifically, upregulation of sensory neuron-specific sodium channels and vanilloid receptors, mechanosensitivity of the dorsal root ganglion, phenotypic modifications of large myelinated axons and sprouting within areas of sensory denervation typically occur. Changes affect the dorsal horn function such as deafferentation hypersensitivity, reduced repetitive firing thresholds, enhanced subthreshold oscillations, activation of intracellular second messenger systems, immediate early gene induction leading to changes in protein synthesis, long-term potentiation of synaptic transmission, and loss of inhibitory mechanisms. Finally, apoptotic neuronal cell death plays an unclear role in regulation of pain sensation, but is measurably affected by nociceptive stimulation [Bolay and Moskowitz, 2002; Zimmermann, 2001].

## Peripheral Mechanisms

Peripheral mechanisms of pain begin with the primary afferent nociceptors that respond to mechanical, thermal, and chemical stimuli [Meyer et al., 1994]. Neuronal subtypes sense and transmit distinct information about actual stimuli. The myelinated Aδ-fibers transmit mechanothermal information (phasic pain with sharp, pricking quality) while unmyelinated C-fiber nociceptors are poly-modal (tonic pain with burning, itching, aching quality) and represent the majority of nociceptors. One class of C-fibers contains neuropeptides such as substance P and calcitonin gene-related peptide and expresses trkA receptors, which have a high affinity for nerve growth factor. These neurons respond to noxious heat and chemicals present during inflammation and synapse with spinal neurons in lamina I and II (outer) that project to higher order pain centers in the brain. The other class of C-fibers has few neuropeptides, expresses a surface carbohydrate group that binds isolectin B4, produces larger magnitude voltage-gated sodium currents, and synapses primarily with local spinal interneurons in the inner portion of lamina II.

While the effects of age on the pain threshold depend on multiple factors such as sensory modality, location in the body, and experimental paradigm, even at the level of the individual nociceptive fibers, age effects show that the system is highly modulated [Chakour et al., 1996; Heft et al., 1996; Lasch et al., 1997]. The pain threshold may be raised in the elderly as indicated by decreased reports of pain with esophageal distension and thermal stimulation to the skin but unaffected in heat/cold pain sensation on the skin of the face or detection of electrical stimulation to the skin. In studies of heat nociception in leg skin, pain intensity ratings were not affected by age [Harkins et al., 1996]. However, in the elderly, slow temporal summation (C-fibers) failed to develop and response times to pain (Aδ-fibers) were delayed. In another study utilizing a compression block of the superficial radial nerve, older adults exhibited an increase in pain threshold consistent with impaired Aδ-fiber function and not that of preserved C-fiber function [Chakour et al., 1996].

Usually, stimulation activates high threshold nociceptors but in conditions of inflammation or nerve injury, neurogenic inflammation occurs with the release of peptides from nociceptive afferents such as substance P and neu-rokinin A [Levine et al., 1993; Woolf and Chong, 1993]. As a result, nerve fibers become more excitable, vascular structures dilate, plasma proteins are extravasated, and cells release a variety of inflammatory mediators (e.g. bradykinin, histamine, arachidonic acid metabolites). When these chemicals alter the response of high threshold nociceptors, peripheral sensitization has occurred. Afterwards, low-intensity stimuli can activate low threshold Aβ-mechanoreceptors and produce allodynia (nonnoxious tactile stimuli perceived as painful). In addition, noxious stimuli typically evoke more pain than normal in a zone of primary hyperalgesia around the site of injury. The decrease in sensory nerve function with age may also be manifested by poor tissue healing which can be reversed with the vasodilation produced by exogenous sensory peptides such as substance P and calcitonin gene-related peptide [Khalil and Helme, 1996; Khalil et al., 1994; Merhi et al., 1998]. High-frequency electrical stimulation of sensory nerves in aged rats produced an increased latency and decreased vasodilation response in injured tissues. The decrease in neurogenic inflammatory response that occurs with age as measured by the axon reflex flare response may be due to decreased substance P content in skin [Helme and McKernan, 1986].

Silent nociceptors are a class of unmyelinated primary afferent neurons that respond only when sensitized by the chemical mediators of inflammation [McMahon and Koltzenburg, 1990]. When local tissues are injured, opioid receptors are produced in the dorsal root ganglion and transported to both the dorsal horn of the spinal cord and peripheral sites where they become 'unmasked' [Stein et al., 1997]. When a nerve is damaged, sodium channels increase in number and appear in novel locations with altered subtype profiles, peptide production increases, the end of the nerve fiber sprouts, sensitivity to mechanical stimulation and noradrenaline increases, and the nerve fires spontaneously and with increased evoked activity [Devor, 1994; Jensen, 2002]. If the mechanically evoked ectopic discharge continues after the end of the stimulus (afterdischarge), then the painful sensation will persist, which is called hyperpathia. Similar changes occur at sites of demyelination and in the dorsal root ganglion of damaged nerves. Sympathetic efferent fibers release prostanoids during inflammation that sensitize primary nociceptive afferents, innervate the dorsal root ganglion, and excite primary afferents at $\alpha$-adrenoceptors [Janig, 1996]. In sympathetically mediated pain states such as complex regional pain syndrome type 1 (reflex sympathetic dystrophy) and type 2 (causalgia), sympathetic efferent activity is decreased but coupled to sensory afferents with increased responsiveness mediated primarily by $\alpha_2$-adrenoceptors that initiate ectopic firing. If this occurs midcourse along the axon, antidromic impulses in C-fibers release various vasoactive peptides from peripheral nociceptor endings such as substance P causing vasodilation, edema, and abnormal growth.

### Dorsal Horn Mechanisms

Further regulation of pain occurs at the level of the spinal synapse. The primary afferent nociceptors terminate in laminae I, II, and V of the dorsal horn [Willis and Coggeshall, 1991]. The second-order neurons project to the thalamus, periaqueductal grey, hypothalamus, amygdala as well as a variety of other higher structures including several regions of the cortex. Rather than a simple relay, these afferents organize the data from the peripheral fibers into a new format. These afferents can be classified into nociceptive-specific/high threshold or wide dynamic range/convergent neurons. The nociceptive-specific neurons are located more superficially in the dorsal horn and respond only to noxious stimuli. In contrast, wide dynamic range neurons are more deeply located and respond to all types of stimuli. Central sensitization can also produce allodynia that occurs when wide dynamic range neurons become hyperexcitable, fire at increased frequency, and produce an abnormally amplified signal usually resulting from strong nociceptive input. The allodynia is manifested in a zone of secondary hyperalgesia in normal tissue adjacent to injured tissue that is due to peripheral input along typically nonnociceptive, thickly myelinated A$\beta$ touch afferents. Local interneurons provide inhibitory modulation.

Sensitization, which is a simple form of learning and synaptic plasticity, can be described as an increased response to neuronal input following noxious stimuli [Baranauskas and Nistri, 1998]. Central sensitization occurs in the dorsal horn, which is the site of action of many neurotransmitters and neuromodulators such as the excitatory amino acids (glutamate, aspartate) and peptides (substance P, tumor necrosis factor-$\alpha$, corticotropin-releasing hormone, galanin) [McLaughlin and Robinson, 2002; Price et al., 1994; Riedel and Neeck, 2001; Zimmerman, 2001]. These act at several receptors including NMDA, kainate, metabotropic glutamate, opioid, neurokinin, $\alpha$-adrenergic, serotonin, adenosine, and $\gamma$-amino-butyric acid (GABA) receptors. GABA is the most abundant inhibitory neurotransmitter in the CNS. Interneurons that utilize GABA are located throughout the spinal cord and along with those that utilize glycine modulate low-threshold afferent inputs. The prolonged activation of non-NMDA receptors (e.g. $\alpha$-amino-3-hydroxy-5-methyl-4-isoxazolepropionic acid) readies the NMDA receptor to produce more long-term changes to the processing of sensory information [Dubner and Ren, 1994; Woolf and Thompson, 1991]. These modifications include wind-up (progressive increases in neuronal activity throughout the stimulus duration), facilitation (magnification and prolongation of the duration of neuron response), action potential threshold reduction, receptive field expansion, oncogene induction, and long-term potentiation (strengthening of synaptic transmission efficacy after activity across the synapse). For example, action potential wind-up is dependent on the rate of membrane potential depolarization during repetitive stimulation and may be due to a number of cell-specific mechanisms including summation of slow excitatory potentials, facilitation of slow calcium channels, and recruitment of NMDA receptor activity [Baranauskas and Nistri, 1998].

Excitatory amino acids such as glutamate are critical for nociceptive processing. A central glutamate transporter system regulates the uptake of endogenous glutamate [Sung et al., 2003]. Chronic constriction nerve injury induces an initial glutamate transporter upregulation that inhibits the development of neuropathic pain behaviors. Subsequent glutamate transporter downregulation was associated with the emergence of thermal hyperalgesia and mechanical allodynia. Glutamate alone acts at both ionotropic and metabotropic types of receptors [Fundytus, 2001; Haberny et al., 2002]. Receptors coupled directly to ion channels are activated by NMDA, α-amino-3-hydroxy-5-methylisoxazole-4-proprionic acid (AMPA), and kainate but metabotropic receptors are G-protein-coupled, interact with intracellular second messengers, and are classified according to structure, signal transduction properties, and receptor pharmacology [Pin and Acher, 2002; Trist, 2000]. In addition, glutamate receptors inhibit or facilitate nociception depending upon their location throughout the CNS. Glutamate also affects aspects of opioid function as well as the broader experience of pain such as depression and anxiety. When calcium enters the cell with the activation of the NMDA receptor, second messengers such as protein kinase C, cGMP, and polyphosphoinosites are generated [Riedel and Neeck, 2001]. Nitric oxide synthase is stimulated and nitric oxide diffuses into neighboring neurons to activate guanylyl cyclase. Adenosine may be a more subtle homeostatic modulator acting through G-protein-coupled receptors that can inhibit or enhance neuronal activity [Ribeiro et al., 2002]. Adenosine receptors inhibit the development and maintenance of central sensitization of spinal dorsal horn neurons.

Approximately 75% of the opioid receptors in the dorsal horn are presynaptic and when stimulated reduce the release of neurotransmitters from primary nociceptive afferents. During inflammation and nerve injury, increased NMDA activity promotes central sensitization and tolerance to opioids, cholecystokinin interferes with opioid analgesia, morphine-3-glucuronide antagonizes opioid analgesia, and presynaptic opioids are lost [Basbaum, 1994; Bennett, 2000]. μ- and δ-opioid receptors can inhibit or potentiate NMDA receptor-mediated activity but κ-opioids antagonize it [Riedel and Neeck, 2001]. Functional inhibition of NMDA receptors may occur as a result of activation at any of the following recognition sites: competitive primary transmitter, strychnine-insensitive glycine (B), polyamine NR2B selective, and phencyclidine [Parsons, 2001]. α-Adrenoceptors are activated by noradrenaline, which has a synergistic effect with opioid receptor agonists and is released by descending inhibitory pathways [Meert and DeKock, 1994]. GABA and glycine tonically inhibit nociception. When activated, GABA$_B$ receptors suppress the presynaptic release of excitatory amino acids from primary afferent terminals whereas GABA$_A$ receptors have postsynaptic actions [Sivilotti and Woolf, 1994].

## Ascending Tract and Descending Inhibition Mechanisms

Second order neurons project to supraspinal structures in the ascending tracts of the contralateral anterolateral spinal cord (spinothalamic, spinoreticular, spinomesencephalic) although not all fibers decussate and a latent ipsilateral pathway is present. The ventroposterior nuclei of the thalamus represent the sensory-discriminative (temporal and spatial) aspects of pain and the medial nuclei are involved with the affective-motivational features of pain. Increased thalamic activity has been associated with acute experimental pain in contrast to chronic pain states, which are associated with decreased thalamic activity on positron emission tomography [Iadarola et al., 1995; Jones et al., 1991]. Most of the other subcortical structures (e.g. basal ganglia, hypothalamus, amygdala, cerebellum) are postulated to function in the transmission of nociception and perception of pain. The basal ganglia receive nociceptive information from multiple afferent sources [Chudler and Dong, 1995]. Positron emission tomography has implicated the nigrostriatal dopaminergic system in central pain modulation with increased D2 receptor binding and presumed decline in endogenous dopamine levels in the putamen of patients with burn mouth syndrome [Hagelberg et al., 2003]. Opioids produce changes in locomotion that correlate with the nigrostriatal release of dopamine [Di Chiara and Imperato, 1988]. $\mu$- and $\delta$-receptor agonists increase dopamine release and locomotion but $\kappa$-receptor agonists decrease dopamine release and locomotion.

The role of the cortical structures in pain and suffering is less well understood. The parietal lobes and somatosensory cortex probably contribute to the sensory-discriminative component and the cingulate cortex with the affective component of pain [Jannetta et al., 1990; Talbot et al., 1991]. Using magnetic resonance spectroscopy, reduced levels of N-acetylaspartate associated with neuronal degeneration have been found in the dorsolateral prefrontal cortex of patients with chronic low back pain and complex regional pain syndrome type I [Grachev et al., 2002]. Pain can be reduced by descending inhibition as first postulated by the gate theory of Melzack and Wall [1965]. Many cerebral structures (e.g. locus ceruleus, nucleus raphe magnus, periaqueductal gray matter, hypothalamus) and neurotransmitters (e.g. endogenous opioids, serotonin, noradrenaline, GABA) contribute to descending inhibition on the dorsal horn and spinal cord [Fields and Basbaum, 1994; Millan, 2002]. Serotonin and dopamine levels have been found to be decreased in studies of nociception in aged rats [Goicoechea et al., 1997]. Corticotropin-releasing hormone can produce analgesia through actions at multiple levels of the nervous system that is independent from the release of $\beta$-endorphin [Lariviere and Melzack, 2000]. Even clonidine can induce analgesia through $\alpha_2$-adrenoceptors that are activated by descending pathways. Treatment modalities involving electrical stimulation (e.g. deep brain stimulation, dorsal column stimulation, transcutaneous electrical nerve stimulation) attempt to activate descending inhibition to decrease chronic pain. Descending facilitory mechanisms arise from medullary sites such as the dorsal reticular nucleus and potentiate nociception through spinal dorsal horn neurons [Lima and Almeida, 2002; Porreca et al., 2002].

## Conclusion

Our current level of understanding of pain is completely inadequate for the development of rational therapeutics. Phantom limb pain is the intense nociceptive experience of the complete absence of neuronal input from an entire field of receptors. It occurs idiopathically in some patients and not in others with identical injuries, and although speculative models exist, it makes clear how little is understood about chronic pain. The modulation of pain at every level of synapse, coupled with the cross talk between pain and affective, executive and cognitive processes complicates our ability to direct care. The good news is the plasticity and integration in the system suggest that ultimately we will be able to intervene and correct disabling symptoms of chronic pain. The few studies that look at improvement suggest that at least some of the changes that occur to upregulate pain are reversible.

Ultimately, the neurobiology of pain is necessary to design rational therapies. Chronic pain treatment has focused on the symptomatic management of existing neuropathic conditions such as postherpetic neuralgia and painful diabetic peripheral neuropathy with encouraging but incomplete success [Dworkin, 2002]. First-line therapies currently include opioids ($\mu$-agonists), antidepressants (monoamine reuptake inhibitors), and anticonvulsants (sodium channel blockers) although many of these agents have multiple pharmacological actions that potentially affect nociception. Continuing neurobiological discoveries generate specific ideas for the development of new pharmacological agents to treat pain mechanistically through modulation of synaptic transmission and membrane excitability with antagonists of sodium channel subtypes, selective NMDA receptor antagonists, adenosine A1 receptor antagonists, nitric oxide synthase inhibitors, and cyclooxygenase-2 inhibitors [Lane, 1997; Lipman, 1996; Parsons, 2001; Ribeiro et al., 2002].

## References

Baranauskas G, Nistri A: Sensitization of pain pathways in the spinal cord: Cellular mechanisms. Prog Neurobiol 1998;54:349–365.

Basbaum AI: Mechanisms of substance P-mediated nociception and opioid-mediated antinociception; in Stanley TH, Ashburn MA (eds): Anesthesiology and Pain Management. Dordrecht, Kluwer Academic, 1994, pp 1–17.

Bennett GJ: Update on the neurophysiology of pain transmission and modulation: Focus on the NMDA-receptor. J Pain Symptom Manage 2000;19(suppl 1):S2–S6.

Besson JM: The neurobiology of pain. Lancet 1999;353:1610–1615.

Bolay H, Moskowitz MA: Mechanisms of pain modulation in chronic syndromes. Neurology 2002; 59(5 suppl 2):S2–S7.

Borsook D: Molecular Neurobiology of Pain, Progress in Pain Research and Management. Seattle, IASP Press, 1997, vol 9.

Cesaro P, Ollat H: Pain and its treatments. Eur Neurol 1997;38:209–215.

Chakour MC, Gibson SJ, Bradbeer M, et al: The effect of age on A$\delta$- and C-fibre thermal pain perception. Pain 1996;64:143–152.

Chudler EH, Dong WK: The role of the basal ganglia in nociception and pain. Pain 1995;60:3–38.

Devor M: The pathophysiology of damaged peripheral nerves; in Wall PD, Melzack R (eds): Textbook of Pain, ed 3. Edinburgh, Churchill Livingstone, 1994, pp 79–100.

Di Chiara G, Imperato A: Opposite effects of $\mu$ and $\kappa$ opiate agonists on dopamine release in the nucleus accumbens and in the dorsal caudate of freely moving rats. J Pharmacol Exp Ther 1988;244: 1067–1080.

Dickenson AH, Matthews EA, Suzuki R: Neurobiology of neuropathic pain: Mode of action of anticonvulsants. Eur J Pain 2002;6(suppl A):51–60.

Dubner R, Ren K: Central mechanisms of thermal and mechanical hyperalgesia following tissue inflammation; in Boivie J, Hansson P, Lindblom U (eds): Touch, Temperature, and Pain in Health and Disease: Mechanisms and Assessments. Seattle, IASP Press, 1994, vol 3, pp 267–277.

Dworkin RH: An overview of neuropathic pain: Syndromes, symptoms, signs, and several mechanisms. Clin J Pain 2002;18:343–349.

Fields HL, Basbaum AI: Central nervous system mechanisms of pain modulation; in Wall PD, Melzack R (eds): Textbook of Pain, ed 3. Edinburgh, Churchill Livingstone, 1994, pp 243–257.

Fundytus ME: Glutamate receptors and nociception: Implications for the drug treatment of pain. CNS Drugs 2001;15:29–58.

Goicoechea C, Ormazabal MJ, Alfaro MJ, et al: Age-related changes in nociception, behavior, and monoamine levels in rats. Gen Pharmacol 1997;28:331–336.

Grachev ID, Thomas PS, Ramachandran TS: Decreased levels of N-acetylaspartate in dorsolateral prefrontal cortex in a case of intractable severe sympathetically mediated chronic pain (complex regional pain syndrome, type I). Brain Cogn 2002;49:102–113.

Haberny KA, Paule MG, Scallet AC, Sistare FD, Lester DS, Hanig JP, Slikker W Jr: Ontogeny of the N-methyl-D-aspartate (NMDA) receptor system and susceptibility to neurotoxicity. Toxicol Sci 2002;68:9–17.

Hagelberg N, Forssell H, Rinne JO, Scheinin H, Taiminen T, Aalto S, Luutonen S, Nagren K, Jaaskelainen S: Striatal dopamine D1 and D2 receptors in burning mouth syndrome. Pain 2003; 101:149–154.

Harkins SW, Davis MD, Bush FM, et al: Suppression of first pain and slow temporal summation of second pain in relation to age. J Gerontol A Biol Sci Med Sci 1996;51:M260–M265.

Heft MW, Cooper BY, O'Brien KK, et al: Aging effects on the perception of noxious and non-noxious thermal stimuli applied to the face. Aging 1996;8:35–41.

Helme RD, McKernan S: Effects of age on the axon reflex response to noxious chemical stimulation. Clin Exp Neurol 1986;22:57–61.

Hunt SP, Mantyh PW: The molecular dynamics of pain control. Nat Rev Neurosci 2001;2:83–91.

Iadarola MJ, Max MB, Berman KF, et al: Unilateral decrease in thalamic activity observed with positron emission tomography in patients with chronic neuropathic pain. Pain 1995;63:55–64.

Janig W: The puzzle of 'reflex sympathetic dystrophy': Mechanisms, hypotheses, open questions; in Janig W, Stanton-Hicks M (eds): Reflex Sympathetic Dystrophy: A Reappraisal. Seattle, IASP Press, 1996, pp 1–24.

Jannetta PJ, Gildenberg PL, Loeser JD, et al: Operations on the brain and brain stem for chronic pain; in Bonica JJ (ed): The Management of Pain. Philadelphia, Lea & Febiger, 1990, vol 2, pp 2082–2103.

Jensen TS: Anticonvulsants in neuropathic pain: Rationale and clinical evidence. Eur J Pain 2002; 6(suppl A):61–68.

Jones AKP, Brown WD, Friston KJ, et al: Cortical and subcortical localization of response to pain in man using positron emission tomography. Proc R Soc Lond B Biol Sci 1991;244:39–44.

Khalil Z, Helme R: Sensory peptides as neuromodulators of wound healing in aged rats. J Gerontol A Biol Sci Med Sci 1996;51:B354–B361.

Khalil Z, Ralevic V, Bassirat M, et al: Effects of ageing on sensory nerve function in rat skin. Brain Res 1994;641:265–272.

Lane NE: Pain management in osteoarthritis: The role of COX-2 inhibitors. J Rheumatol 1997;24 (suppl 49):20–24.

Lariviere WR, Melzack R: The role of corticotropin-releasing factor in pain and analgesia. Pain 2000; 84:1–12.

Lasch H, Castell DO, Castell JA: Evidence for diminished visceral pain with aging: Studies using graded intraesophageal balloon distension. Am J Physiol 1997;272:G1–G3.

Levine JD, Fields HL, Basbaum AI: Peptides and the primary afferent nociceptor. J Neurosci 1993;13: 2273–2286.

Lima D, Almeida A: The medullary dorsal reticular nucleus as a pronociceptive center of the pain control system. Prog Neurobiol 2002;66:81–108.

Lipman AG: Analgesic drugs for neuropathic and sympathetically maintained pain. Clin Geriatr Med 1996;12:501–515.

McLaughlin PJ, Robinson JK: Galanin: Involvement in Behavior and Neuropathology, and Therapeutic Potential. Drug News Perspect 2002;15:647–653.

McMahon S, Koltzenburg M: The changing role of primary afferent neurones in pain. Pain 1990;43: 269–272.

Meert TF, DeKock M: Potentiation of the analgesic properties of fentanyl-like opioids with alpha2-adrenoceptor agonists in rats. Anesthesiology 1994;81:677–688.

Melzack R, Wall PD: Pain mechanisms: A new theory. Science 1965;150:971–979.

Merhi M, Helme RD, Khalil Z: Age-related changes in sympathetic modulation of sensory nerve activity in rat skin. Inflamm Res 1998;47:239–244.

Meyer RA, Campbell JN, Raja SN: Peripheral neural mechanisms of nociception; in Wall PD, Melzack R (eds): Textbook of Pain, ed 3. Edinburgh, Churchill Livingstone, 1994, pp 13–44.

Millan MJ: Descending control of pain. Prog Neurobiol 2002;66:355–474.

Parsons CG: NMDA receptors as targets for drug action in neuropathic pain. Eur J Pharmacol 2001; 429:71–78.

Pin JP, Acher F: The metabotropic glutamate receptors: Structure, activation mechanism and pharmacology. Curr Drug Target CNS Neurol Disord 2002;1:297–317.

Porreca F, Ossipov MH, Gebhart GF: Chronic pain and medullary descending facilitation. Trends Neurosci 2002;25:319–325.

Price DD, Mao JR, Mayer DJ: Central neural mechanisms of normal and abnormal pain states; in Fields HL, Liebeskind JC (eds): Pharmacological Approaches to the Treatment of Chronic Pain: New Concepts and Critical Issues. Progress in Pain Research and Management. Seattle, IASP Press, 1994, vol 1, pp 61–84.

Price DD: Psychological and neural mechanisms of the affective dimension of pain. Science 2000;288: 1769–1772.

Ribeiro JA, Sebastiao AM, de Mendonca A: Adenosine receptors in the nervous system: Pathophysiological implications. Prog Neurobiol 2002;68:377–392.

Riedel W, Neeck G: Nociception, pain, and antinociception: Current concepts. Z Rheumatol 2001;60: 404–415.

Siddal PJ, Cousins MJ: Pain mechanisms and management: An update. Clin Exp Pharmacol Physiol 1995;22:679–688.

Siddal PJ, Cousins MJ: Introduction to pain mechanisms. Implications for neural blockade; in Cousins MJ, Bridenbaugh PO (eds): Neural Blockade in Clinical Anesthesia and Management of Pain, ed 3. Philadelphia, Lippincott-Raven, 1998, pp 675–713.

Sivilotti L, Woolf CJ: The contribution of GABA-A and glycine receptors to central sensitization: Disinhibition and touch-evoked allodynia in the spinal cord. J Neurophysiol 1994;72:169–179.

Stein C, Schafer M, Cabot PJ, et al: Opioids and inflammation; in Borsook D (ed): Molecular Neurobiology of Pain, Progress in Pain Research and Management. Seattle, IASP Press, 1997, vol 9, pp 25–43.

Sung B, Lim G, Mao J: Altered expression and uptake activity of spinal glutamate transporters after nerve injury contribute to the pathogenesis of neuropathic pain in rats. J Neurosci 2003;23: 2899–2910.

Talbot JD, Marrett S, Evans AC, et al: Multiple representations of pain in human cerebral cortex. Science 1991;251:1355–1358.

Trist DG: Excitatory amino acid agonists and antagonists: Pharmacology and therapeutic applications. Pharm Acta Helv 2000;74:221–229.

Wall PD, Melzack R: Textbook of Pain, ed 3. Edinburgh, Churchill Livingstone, 1994.

Willis WD, Coggeshall RE: Sensory Mechanisms of the Spinal Cord. New York, Plenum Press, 1991.

Woolf CJ, Chong MS: Pre-emptive analgesia-treating postoperative pain by preventing the establishment of central sensitization. Anesth Analg 1993;77:362–379.

Woolf CJ, Thompson SWN: The induction and maintenance of central sensitization is dependent on N-methyl-*D*-aspartic acid receptor activation; implications for the treatment of post-injury pain hypersensitivity states. Pain 1991;44:293–299.

Zimmermann M: Pathobiology of neuropathic pain. Eur J Pharmacol 2001;429:23–37.

Michael R. Clark, MD, MPH
Associate Professor and Director, Adolf Meyer Chronic Pain Treatment Programs
Department of Psychiatry and Behavioral Sciences, Johns Hopkins Medical Institutions
Osler 320, 600 North Wolfe Street, Baltimore, MD 21287–5371 (USA)
Tel. +1 410 955 2126, Fax +1 410 614 8760, E-Mail mrclark@jhmi.edu

Clark MR, Treisman GJ (eds): Pain and Depression. An Interdisciplinary Patient-Centered
Approach. Adv Psychosom Med. Basel, Karger, 2004, vol 25, pp 89–101

..........................

# Complex Regional Pain Syndrome: Diagnostic Controversies, Psychological Dysfunction, and Emerging Concepts

*Theodore S. Grabow, Paul J. Christo, Srinivasa N. Raja*

Division of Pain Medicine, Department of Anesthesiology and Critical Care
Medicine, Johns Hopkins University School of Medicine, Baltimore, Md., USA

## Abstract

Complex regional pain syndromes (CRPS) types I and II are neuropathic pain disorders
that involve dysfunction of the peripheral and central nervous system. CRPS type I and type II
were known formerly as reflex sympathetic dystrophy and causalgia, respectively. Most experts
believe that a multidisciplinary approach including pharmacotherapy, physiotherapy, and psychotherapy is warranted. Historically, there has been considerable controversy regarding this
disease entity. In particular, the precise mechanism of the sympathetic dysfunction as well as
the nature of the psychological dysfunction commonly observed in patients with CRPS has
been the subject of considerable debate. Current strides in our understanding of the pathophysiology of this disease have improved treatment options.

## Introduction

Complex regional pain syndrome (CRPS) type I and type II, formerly
known as reflex sympathetic dystrophy (RSD) and causalgia, respectively, are
neuropathic pain disorders likely involving dysfunction of both the peripheral
and central nervous system (CNS). The pathophysiology is poorly understood
and treatments often are directed at managing the signs and symptoms of
disease. A significant number of patients exhibit comorbid psychological
dysfunction which has led some clinicians to believe incorrectly that CRPS is
entirely a psychiatric disease. Animal research has improved our mechanistic
understanding of neuropathic pain and this awareness may facilitate our understanding of CRPS (particularly CRPS type II). Recent clinical investigation has

resulted in an improved understanding of the biological dysfunction observed in patients with CRPS. This review will (1) summarize the historical arguments and controversy surrounding the disease, (2) describe the psychological dysfunction often observed in patients with CRPS, and (3) discuss recent trends in the neurobiological understanding of CRPS.

## CRPS Controversy and Misunderstanding

### CRPS History

Several authors have questioned the validity of CRPS type I as an actual organically based neurological disease and have doubted the involvement of the sympathetic nervous system in the maintenance of the pain. Many aspects of the disease, including nomenclature, etiopathogenesis, diagnosis, and treatment have generated considerable controversy. As a result, CRPS type I (RSD) has been considered by some experts an expression of somatoform disease and therefore has been designated as pseudoneuropathy of psychogenic origin. A brief discussion of several of these arguments is warranted.

### Nomenclature

Causalgia was first described in 1864 as a distinct disease entity by Silas Weir Mitchell who noted extreme pain, autonomic abnormalities, trophic changes, and involuntary movements in Civil War soldiers who suffered from traumatic injury to peripheral nerves. Rene Leriche later postulated in 1916 that the sympathetic nervous system was involved in pain states involving major tissue or nerve injury. The term RSD was coined nearly half a century later in 1946 by J.A. Evans to describe patients who exhibited causalgia-like symptoms but without evidence of major tissue or nerve injury. Several other terms have been used to describe this disease such as minor causalgia, algodystrophy, shoulder-hand syndrome, posttraumatic dystrophy, and Sudeck's atrophy. In general, the disease was given different names based on the personal assumptions, frame of reference, institutional background, or country of origin of the investigators who were describing the disease process.

In 1994, a task force commissioned by the International Association for the Study of Pain (IASP) introduced the present day descriptive terminology to standardize the nomenclature, remove obsolete mechanistic understandings, and improve disease recognition. Until this time, scholars had argued that the term RSD erroneously implied an underlying 'reflexive' mechanism presumably related to aberrant function (ex. hyperactivity) of the sympathetic nervous system that if left untreated would inevitably lead to permanent dystrophic change. Today, most authorities recognize that sympathetic 'overactivity' is not observed and that sympathetic dysfunction and dystrophic changes occur only in a subset of patients with CRPS. Furthermore, certain therapies specifically aimed at the sympathetic nervous system may be unwarranted [1, 2]. Despite the efforts of the IASP, many clinicians are unfamiliar with modern taxonomy and the majority of contemporary investigators fail to utilize the diagnostic criteria proposed by the IASP [3, 4].

*Diagnosis*

According to the IASP, the diagnosis of CRPS requires (1) an initiating noxious event or cause of immobilization, (2) continuing pain, allodynia, or hyperalgesia disproportionate to any inciting event, (3) evidence at some time of edema, changes in skin blood flow, or abnormal sudomotor activity, and (4) the exclusion of a medical condition that would otherwise account for the degree of pain and dysfunction. The presence of an initiating noxious event or cause of immobilization was not required according to the original publication by the IASP in 1994; however, this statement was omitted from the more widely available and Medline-indexed summary statement from the consensus meeting published in 1995 [5]. Importantly, a precipitating inciting event may not be detected in approximately 10% of patients with CRPS [6]. This definition is entirely descriptive and does not imply etiology nor specific pathophysiology. This lack of mechanism-based specificity in the proposed diagnostic criteria has detracted somewhat from its universal acceptance by the scientific community.

*Etiopathogenesis*

Patients with CRPS exhibit signs of emotional duress and psychological dysfunction. Consequently, it was tempting for early investigators to conclude that much of the pain and symptomatology was the result of untreated psychiatric disease or caused by exaggerated sympathoarousal secondary to underlying stress. The term RSD helped to maintain this cause and effect link between the sympathetic nervous system and the pain. As a result, many patients underwent therapies designed to mitigate sympathetic nervous system function. Today, there is convincing evidence in animals and humans that nerve injury and tissue inflammation may be associated with aberrant functioning of the sympathetic nervous system [7] (table 1). Despite this link, the pathophysiology of CRPS is incompletely understood and several mechanisms may be operational simultaneously. Furthermore, it is commonly recognized that only a subset of patients with CRPS have sympathetically maintained pain, which is defined as pain that is modulated by sympathetic block or pharmacological antagonism of α-adrenoceptor function.

***Table 1.*** Sympathetic nervous system involvement after nerve injury and inflammation

| | |
|---|---|
| Animal studies | Sprouting of sympathetic fibers in neuroma and DRG |
| | Upregulation of adrenoceptors in neuroma and DRG |
| | Sympathetic fiber migration into denervated skin |
| | Increase afferent, neuroma, and DRG sensitivity to NE, sympathetic stimulation, and stress; effects are decreased by α-adrenergic antagonists |
| | Decrease in allodynia or hyperalgesia after chemical or surgical sympathectomy |
| | NE rekindles pain behavior after sympathectomy |
| | Increase in pain behaviors with NE injection or during stress |
| Human studies | Sympathetic sprouting in DRG [29] |
| | Increase in adrenoceptors in skin [30] |
| | Topical $\alpha_2$-adrenoceptor agonists decrease pain in the affected region |
| | Chemical or surgical sympathectomy decreases pain |
| | Subcutaneous injection of NE or sympathetic stimulation rekindles pain after sympathectomy |
| | Increase in reported pain with stress or NE [31] |
| | Chemically mediated allodynia and hyperalgesia are decreased by adrenergic antagonists and increased by NE [32] |
| | Increase in pain and hyperalgesia after physiological activation of the sympathetic nervous system [35] |

Selected references provided [for further details, see 7].

## Psychological Dysfunction

### Psychiatric Comorbid Conditions in Chronic Pain

Chronic pain patients frequently have associated comorbid psychiatric disease [8]. When ranked from most frequent to least frequent, the following comorbid conditions likely are associated more with chronic pain patients than with the general population: affective disorders (depression), psychoactive substance use-related disorders, somatoform disorders, and anxiety disorders. Moreover, a significant number of chronic pain patients may have more than one axis I psychiatric comorbidity. Psychiatric comorbidities can have a negative impact on chronic pain and functional status. In addition, there are a group of conditions commonly observed in chronic pain patients that are not necessarily psychiatric in nature, which in addition do not satisfy formal Diagnostic and Statistical Manual (DSM) criteria. These observations include such things as pain behaviors, sleep disturbance, somatization, nonorganic physical findings, and impaired functional status out of proportion to physician expectations based on objective findings [8]. The prognostic implications of these conditions is unknown.

### Psychiatric Disease in CRPS

Patients with CRPS commonly suffer from psychological dysfunction. In fact, patients with CRPS experience a significant amount of depression, anxiety, and phobia. However, attempts to establish a unique 'CRPS personality' have been unsuccessful. In general, early studies lacked validity due to various flaws in methodological design. For example, studies failed to examine premorbid personality data, study investigators used heterogenous definitions of psychiatric terminology, and psychometric instruments had not been 'normed' on pain populations [9]. Nevertheless, reported prevalence of psychiatric disorders in patients with CRPS ranges from 18 to 64% [10]. Psychological examination using the Structured Clinical Interview (SCID) of the DSM-IV demonstrates a high frequency of affective disorder (46%), anxiety disorder (27%), and substance abuse disorder (14%) in patients with CRPS [11]. However, the prevalence of psychiatric disorders in patients with CRPS may not be much different from chronic pain patients in general. For example, the prevalence of major depression (1.5–54.5%), anxiety disorders (7–62.5%), and substance abuse disorders (3.2–18.9%) in chronic pain patients is reported in similar rates as CRPS patients [8]. Finally, Bruehl and Carlson [10] reviewed data strictly from studies which used the Minnesota Multiphasic Personality Inventory (MMPI) and concluded that patients with CRPS, like patients with chronic pain in general, are somatically preoccupied, depressed, and use repression as a psychological defense mechanism.

There has been historical debate whether chronic pain or psychiatric illness is the primary process. The reciprocal relationship between pain and psychological dysfunction in patients with CRPS is evident from a recent study of daily diaries which demonstrated that yesterday's depressed mood contributed to today's increased pain and that yesterday's pain also contributed to today's depression, anxiety, and anger [12]. Several literature reviews have examined whether psychological dysfunction was the cause or effect of CRPS [9, 10, 13]. In general, the majority of historical studies suffered from flaws in methodology such as lack of consistent and homogenous diagnostic groups, lack of control groups and significant statistical tests, lack of objective measures of psychological disease, poorly defined behavioral criteria, and incorrect use of psychiatric or psychological terminology [13]. As a result, Lynch [13] concluded there is no valid evidence that certain personality traits or psychological factors predispose one to the development of CRPS. Similarly, due to the methodological weakness of the literature, Bruehl and Carlson [10] concluded there is insufficient data to draw meaningful conclusions whether or not preexisting psychological factors predispose to the development of CRPS.

In summary, most authors have concluded that comorbid psychological disease in patients with CRPS is a consequence of the chronic pain rather than its cause [9, 13]. Furthermore, there is no evidence that individuals with certain personality types are predisposed to developing CRPS. Finally, there are no consistent psychological differences between CRPS and non-CRPS pain patients [14–22] (table 2).

### Factitious Disorder

The overall prevalence of factitious disorder in chronic pain patients is between 0.14 and 2% [8]. Patients with conversion disorder and factitious illness may have similar clinical presentation to patients with CRPS. In fact, certain sensory signs (ex. nonanatomical and expansive areas of hypoesthesia or hyperalgesia with normal peripheral sensory nerve conduction or somatosensory evoked potentials) or features (ex. normalization of hypoesthesia by nerve blocks) identified in patients with CRPS type I likely are psychogenic in origin. Moreover, neurophysiological investigation suggests that certain positive motor signs (dystonia, tremors, spasms, irregular jerks) identified in patients with CRPS type I are in fact psychogenic in origin and represent pseudoneurological illness [23].

### Strain and Distress in Caregivers

Caregivers of patients with CRPS experience significant levels of strain and susceptibility to depression measured by the Caregiver Strain Index (CSI) and General Health Questionnaire-12 (GHQ-12), respectively [24]. Caregiver health can have a significant impact on recipient care. Thus, physicians should not only implement psychosocial interventions directed at patients but also at caregivers of patients with CRPS.

### Other Issues (Legal, Disability)

Allen et al. [25] recently performed a retrospective chart review of the epidemiology of CRPS. They reported that 54% of patients had a worker compensation claim and that 17% had a lawsuit related to the CRPS. The effect of litigation on pain severity and clinical outcomes for patients with CRPS is unknown.

### Neglect-Like Symptoms

Patients with CRPS often display signs of motor dysfunction that appear to be related to voluntary guarding in order to avoid exacerbation of pain.

***Table 2.*** Psychological comparisons of CRPS and chronic pain patients

| Study | Comparison group | Psychological measure(s) | Conclusion |
|---|---|---|---|
| Haddox et al., 1988 [14] | Painful radiculopathy | STAI, DPQ, McGill Pain Questionnaire | No differences |
| Zuchinni et al., 1989 [15] | Nerve lesion | MMPI | No differences |
| DeGood et al., 1993 [16] | Chronic low back pain | SCL-90R | Less distress but higher pain-related disability and pain scores in CRPS |
| Nelson and Novy, 1996 [17] | Myofascial pain syndrome | MMPI | Less psychological dysfunction, less pain medication, more employment disruption, and more worker's compensation in CRPS |
| Bruehl et al., 1996 [18] | Chronic low back pain and chronic limb pain | McGill Pain Questionnaire, CSQ, BSI | More emotional distress, positive pain coping behavior, and somatization in CRPS |
| Ciccone et al., 1997 [19] | Chronic low back pain and chronic radiculopathy | BDI, CSAQ, SIP | No differences except greater disability days in CRPS and low back pain |
| Geertzen et al., 1998 [20] | Hand pathology | SCL-90, STAI | More depression in female patients and more anxiety in male patients with CRPS |
| Monti et al., 1998 [21] | Chronic low back pain | SCID, SCID II | No differences |
| Van der Laan et al., 1999 [22] | CRPS with dystonia and chronic Rehab population | SCL-90R | No differences except more insomnia and less somatization in CRPS-dystonia group |

STAI = State-Trait Anxiety Inventory; DPQ = Dartmount Pain Questionnaire; SCL-90R = System Checklist-90 Revised; CSQ = Coping Strategies Questionnaire; BSI = Brief System Inventory; BDI = Beck Depression Inventory; CSAQ = Cognitive-Somatic Anxiety Questionnaire; SIP = Sickness Impact Profile.

However, recent evidence suggests that motor dysfunction may be related to neglect-like symptoms (i.e. cognitive neglect, motor neglect) in a subset of patients with CRPS [26]. Of note, self-reported motor dysfunction is the second most commonly reported group of symptoms after sensory dysfunction in patients with CRPS [27].

*Quality of Life*

A pilot study demonstrated substantial interference with quality of life measured by modified Brief Pain Inventory (mBPI) as well as significant sleep disturbance in patients with CRPS [27].

*Stressful Life Events*

Stressful life events were more common in patients with CRPS than in a control group of patients with hand pathology measured by the Social Readjustment Rating Scale (SRRS) [20]. However, these authors concluded that there was no direct causal relationship between these stressful life events or any underlying psychological dysfunction (measured by SCL-90) and the onset of CRPS. In a retrospective study, Geertzen et al. [28] concluded that stressful life events and psychological dysfunction, measured by the SRRS and RAND 36-item Health Survey (RAND-36), respectively, already existed at the time of diagnosis of CRPS and did not result from CRPS.

## Recent Trends

*Sympathetic Nervous System*

Classical teaching suggested that the sympathetic nervous system was the cause of pain or maintained the pain in patients with CRPS. Although authors recognized that certain patients with CRPS displayed signs of sympathetic nervous system dysfunction, many were reluctant to concede that pain was caused by the aberrant functioning of the sympathetic nervous system. Contemporary understanding suggests that the sympathetic nervous system not only may be dysfunctional but also that it can modulate the pain experience in patients with CRPS. In addition, the dysfunction of the sympathetic nervous system may be both peripheral and central in origin which may account for the complex and widespread symptomatology observed in patients with CRPS. A brief review of pertinent studies is warranted.

*Sympathetic Nervous System and Pain*

In animals, there is overwhelming evidence that nerve injury and inflammation can result in functional coupling between the sympathetic efferent and primary sensory afferent neurons within the peripheral nervous system [7]. The site of this aberrant sympathetic-sensory coupling involves the dorsal root ganglia (DRG), the area of injury itself (i.e. neuroma site), or within the tissue innervated by the injured nerve.

Several of these correlates exist in humans and these findings have been summarized in recent reviews [7]. For example, peripheral nerve injury results in sympathetic sprouting and functional coupling between sympathetic efferent and primary sensory afferent neurons in the DRG [29]. An increase of $\alpha_1$-adrenoceptors has been observed in the hyperalgesic skin of patients with CRPS type I [30]. Patients with CRPS type I have decreased sympathetic outflow but increased $\alpha$-adrenergic responsiveness in the affected limbs suggesting adrenergic supersensitivity. This supersensitivity is reversed when CRPS symptoms resolve. Pharmacological or surgical sympathectomy can decrease pain in patients with CRPS and patients with neuropathic pain report increased pain during stress or after intradermal injection of a physiological dose of norepinephrine (NE) [31]. In addition, injection of NE can rekindle pain and mechanical hyperalgesia in patients who have had a previous sympathetic block. Finally, inflammatory pain and hyperalgesia produced by topical capsaicin is decreased by $\alpha_1$-adrenoceptor antagonists and increased by NE [32].

Despite this evidence, systematic reviews have failed to demonstrate the efficacy of therapies designed to inhibit sympathetic function and question their utility [1, 2]. In fact, some investigators have challenged the validity of pharmacological tests to establish the diagnosis of sympathetically maintained pain. The interpretation of results from diagnostic and prognostic nerve blocks for chronic pain can be challenging even for clinicians with considerable expertise [33].

Recent studies have examined the effect of the natural stimulation of the subject's own sympathetic nervous system on spontaneous pain and hyperalgesia rather than the effect of pharmacological treatment such as sympathetic block or injection of NE. Sympathetic arousal increased pain and vasoconstriction in the affected extremity of patients with CRPS types I and II [34]. Also, sympathetic activation increased spontaneous pain and spatial distribution of mechanical hyperalgesia in patients with CRPS type I who have sympathetically maintained pain [35]. These two investigations were the first to demonstrate that physiological activation of the sympathetic nervous system can modulate the pain experience in humans through endogenous release of NE from sympathetic nerve endings. These findings provide evidence in support of the concept of sympathetically maintained pain, or pain as the result of sympathetic efferent activity.

*Sympathetic Nervous System Dysfunction*
In the acute stage of CRPS type I, there is complete functional loss of cutaneous sympathetic vasoconstrictor activity as well as decreased venous plasma levels of NE (presumably secondary to decreased postganglionic release from sympathetic terminals) confined to the affected extremity [36]. This autonomic impairment may recover within weeks and likely reflects dysfunction within the CNS. During chronic CRPS, sympathetic vasoconstrictor neurons are still inhibited, but adrenoceptor supersensitivity in vascular tissue results in ongoing

vasoconstriction and subsequent cold skin. These vascular abnormalities are dynamic and more pronounced when examined over the entire range of the thermoregulatory cycle [37].

Patients with acute CRPS type I also demonstrate α-adrenergic supersensitivity of sudomotor nerves that is reversible with disease progression [38]. Unilateral disturbances in sudomotor function determined by quantitative sudomotor axon reflex test (QSART) and thermoregulatory sweat test (TST) also have been reported in patients with chronic CRPS [39].

*Sensory Dysfunction*

Sensory disturbances are common in patients with CRPS types I and II and predominantly consist of hyperalgesia, allodynia, and spontaneous pain [6]. Quantitative sensory testing (QST) demonstrates an increase in warm perception thresholds and a decrease of cold pain thresholds in patients with CRPS types I and II [40]. Sensory impairments frequently extend beyond the affected area and may involve quadratic or hemilateral regions of the body [41].

*Motor Dysfunction*

Motor disturbances are prevalent in patients with CRPS types I and II [6] and are independent of sensory and autonomic complaints [40]. The most frequently described motor disturbance is loss of function of the affected extremity. Detailed neurological examination may detect objective evidence of isolated motor weakness, muscle atrophy, tremor, dystonia, or ataxia. Furthermore, electrodiagnostic tests such as electromyography and nerve conduction velocity can be used to document muscle and large fiber abnormalities, respectively. Decrease in active range of motion can be assessed by goniometer. Similarly, muscle power can be assessed by measuring grip force strength or by manual muscle testing. More complex motor tasks can be measured by kinematic analysis. A recent study has demonstrated neurophysiological evidence of impairment of central sensorimotor integration in patients with CRPS type I [42]. These motor deficits may be secondary to abnormal integration of visual and sensory inputs to the parietal cortex [43].

*CNS Dysfunction*

Evidence suggests that certain autonomic, motor, and sensory disturbances in patients with CRPS are caused by dysfunction within the CNS whereas certain aspects of the pain itself may be related to aberrant peripheral mechanisms. Potential peripheral and central mechanisms are described elsewhere [7, 44]. Occasionally, dysfunction of the sensory, motor, or autonomic nervous system may involve bilateral structures after unilateral nerve or tissue injury [45]. In addition, several investigators have described CNS abnormalities by fMRI,

MRS, or SPECT. Recent investigation suggests that patients with CRPS may develop functional or structural cortical reorganization and change in central representation of sensory maps. However, it is unclear whether these abnormalities are a result of the chronic pain or whether they represent specific regions of primary dysfunction within the CNS.

### Treatment Algorithm for CRPS

The therapeutic strategy for patients with CRPS involves the concurrent utilization of pharmaco-, physio-, and psychotherapy. However, randomized controlled trials (RCTs) investigating the impact of psychological interventions on homogenous groups of patients with neuropathic pain, including patients with CRPS, have not been undertaken [46]. Nevertheless, principles derived from operant and cognitive behavior theory are useful to treat chronic pain patients in general and these strategies should be used for patients with CRPS. The goal of pharmacological therapy is to reduce pain in order to facilitate functional restoration. In general, medications that are effective for the treatment of neuropathic pain are used for patients with CRPS. The goal of physical therapy is to improve functional status. In general, desensitization and physical rehabilitation cannot proceed without adequate pain control. Most authorities believe that active participation in physical therapy is instrumental for improvement in patients with CRPS. To date, only the short-term efficacy of physical therapy has been demonstrated by an RCT specifically for patients with CRPS [47]. Recent RCTs have demonstrated the efficacy of spinal cord stimulation for the treatment of pain and intrathecal baclofen for the treatment of dystonia in patients with CRPS. The use of these interventional techniques should be considered in the treatment algorithm when other therapies have failed. A summary of current therapeutic strategies for CRPS has been published [48].

### Acknowledgment

This study was supported in part by NIH Grant NS-26363 (SNR).

### References

1 Perez RS, Kwakkel G, Zuurmond WW, de Lange JJ: Treatment of reflex sympathetic dystrophy (CRPS type 1): A research synthesis of 21 randomized clinical trials. J Pain Symptom Manage 2001;21:511–526.
2 Cepeda MS, Lau J, Carr DB: Defining the therapeutic role of local anesthetic sympathetic blockade in complex regional pain syndrome: A narrative and systematic review. Clin J Pain 2002;18: 216–233.
3 Reinders MF, Geertzen JH, Dijkstra PU: Complex regional pain syndrome type I: Use of the International Association for the Study of Pain diagnostic criteria defined in 1994. Clin J Pain 2002;18:207–215.

4    van de Beek WJ, Schwartzman RJ, van Nes SI, Delhaas EM, van Hilten JJ: Diagnostic criteria used in studies of reflex sympathetic dystrophy. Neurology 2002;58:522–526.

5    Stanton-Hicks M, Janig W, Hassenbusch S, Haddox JD, Boas R, Wilson P: Reflex sympathetic dystrophy: Changing concepts and taxonomy. Pain 1995;63:127–133.

6    Veldman PH, Reynen HM, Arntz IE, Goris RJ: Signs and symptoms of reflex sympathetic dystrophy: Prospective study of 829 patients. Lancet 1993;342:1012–1016.

7    Baron R, Levine JD, Fields HL: Causalgia and reflex sympathetic dystrophy: Does the sympathetic nervous system contribute to the generation of pain? Muscle Nerve 1999;22:678–695.

8    Fishbain DA: Approaches to treatment decisions for psychiatric comorbidity in the management of the chronic pain patient. Med Clin North AM 1999;83:737–760.

9    Haddox JD: Psychological aspects of reflex sympathetic dystrophy; in Stanton-Hicks M (ed): Pain and the Sympathetic Nervous System. Boston, Kluwer Academic, 1990, pp 207–224.

10   Bruehl S, Carlson CR: Predisposing psychological factors in the development of reflex sympathetic dystrophy. A review of the empiric evidence. Clin J Pain 1992;8:287–299.

11   Rommel O, Malin JP, Zenz M, Janig W: Quantitative sensory testing, neurophysiological and psychological examination in patients with complex regional pain syndrome and hemisensory deficits. Pain 2001;93:279–293.

12   Feldman SI, Downey G, Schaffer-Neitz R: Pain, negative mood, and perceived support in chronic pain patients: A daily diary study of people with reflex sympathetic dystrophy syndrome. J Consult Clin Psychol 1999;67:776–785.

13   Lynch ME: Psychological aspects of reflex sympathetic dystrophy: A review of the adult and paediatric literature. Pain 1992;49:337–347.

14   Haddox JD, Abram SE, Hopwood MH: Comparison of psychometric data in RSD and radiculopathy. Reg Anesth 1988;13:27.

15   Zucchini M, Alberti G, Moretti MP: Algodystrophy and related psychological features. Funct Neurol 1989;4:153–156.

16   DeGood DE, Cundiff GW, Adams LE, Shutty MS Jr: A psychosocial and behavioral comparison of reflex sympathetic dystrophy, low back pain, and headache patients. Pain 1993;54:317–322.

17   Nelson DV, Novy DM: Psychological characteristics of reflex sympathetic dystrophy versus myofascial pain syndromes. Reg Anesth 1996;21:202–208.

18   Bruehl S, Husfeldt B, Lubenow TR, Nath H, Ivankovich AD: Psychological differences between reflex sympathetic dystrophy and non-RSD chronic pain patients. Pain 1996;67:107–114.

19   Ciccone DS, Bandilla EB, Wu W: Psychological dysfunction in patients with reflex sympathetic dystrophy. Pain 1997;71:323–333.

20   Geertzen JH, de Bruijn-Kofman AT, de Bruijn HP, van de Wiel HB, Dijkstra PU: Stressful life events and psychological dysfunction in complex regional pain syndrome type I. Clin J Pain 1998; 14:143–147.

21   Monti DA, Herring CL, Schwartzman RJ, Marchese M: Personality assessment of patients with complex regional pain syndrome type I. Clin J Pain 1998;14:295–302.

22   van der Laan L, van Spaendonck K, Horstink MW, Goris RJ: The Symptom Checklist-90 Revised questionnaire: No psychological profiles in complex regional pain syndrome-dystonia. J Pain Symptom Manage 1999;17:357–362.

23   Verdugo RJ, Ochoa JL: Abnormal movements in complex regional pain syndrome: Assessment of their nature. Muscle Nerve 2000;23:198–205.

24   Blake H: Strain and psychological distress among informal supporters of reflex sympathetic dystrophy patients. Disabil Rehabil 2000;22:827–832.

25   Allen G, Galer BS, Schwartz L: Epidemiology of complex regional pain syndrome: A retrospective chart review of 134 patients. Pain 1999;80:539–544.

26   Galer BS, Jensen M: Neglect-like symptoms in complex regional pain syndrome: Results of a self-administered survey. J Pain Symptom Manage 1999;18:213–217.

27   Galer BS, Henderson J, Perander J, Jensen MP: Course of symptoms and quality of life measurements in complex regional pain syndrome: A pilot survey. J Pain Symptom Manage 2000;20:286–292.

28   Geertzen JH, Dijkstra PU, Groothoff JW, ten Duis HJ, Eisma WH: Reflex sympathetic dystrophy of the upper extremity – A 5.5 year follow-up. II. Social life events, general health and changes in occupation. Acta Orthop Scand Suppl 1998;279:19–23.

29  Shinder V, Govrin-Lippman R, Cohen S, Belenky M, Ilin P, Fried K, Wilkinson HA, Devor M: Structural basis of sympathetic-sensory coupling in rat and human dorsal root ganglia following peripheral nerve injury. J Neurocytol 1999;28:743–761.

30  Drummond PD, Skipworth S, Finch PM: Alpha 1-adrenoceptors in normal and hyperalgesic human skin. Clin Sci (Lond) 1996;91:73–77.

31  Ali Z, Raja SN, Wesselmann U, Fuchs PN, Meyer RA, Campbell JN: Intradermal injection of nor-epinephrine evokes pain in patients with sympathetically maintained pain. Pain 2000;88:161–168.

32  Drummond PD: Noradrenaline increases hyperalgesia to heat in skin sensitized by capsaicin. Pain 1995;60:311–315.

33  Hogan QH, Abram SE: Neural blockade for diagnosis and prognosis. A review. Anesthesiology 1997;86:216–241.

34  Drummond PD, Finch PM, Skipworth S, Blockey P: Pain increases during sympathetic arousal in patients with complex regional pain syndrome. Neurology 2001;57:1296–1303.

35  Baron R, Schattschneider J, Binder A, Siebrecht D, Wasner G: Relation between sympathetic vasoconstrictor activity and pain and hyperalgesia in complex regional pain syndromes: A case-control study. Lancet 2002;359:1655–1660.

36  Wasner G, Heckmann K, Maier C, Baron R: Vascular abnormalities in acute reflex sympathetic dystrophy (CRPS I): Complete inhibition of sympathetic nerve activity with recovery. Arch Neurol 1999;56:613–620.

37  Wasner G, Schattschneider J, Heckmann K, Maier C, Baron R: Vascular abnormalities in reflex sympathetic dystrophy (CRPS I): Mechanisms and diagnostic value. Brain 2001;124:387–399.

38  Chemali KR, Gorodeski R, Chelimsky TC: Alpha-adrenergic supersensitivity of the sudomotor nerve in complex regional pain syndrome. Ann Neurol 2001;49:453–459.

39  Birklein F, Riedl B, Claus D, Neundorfer B: Pattern of autonomic dysfunction in time course of complex regional pain syndrome. Clin Auton Res 1998;8:79–85.

40  Birklein F, Riedl B, Sieweke N, Weber M, Neundorfer B: Neurological findings in complex regional pain syndromes – Analysis of 145 cases. Acta Neurol Scand 2000;101:262–269.

41  Rommel O, Gehling M, Dertwinkel R, Witscher K, Zenz M, Malin JP, Janig W: Hemisensory impairment in patients with complex regional pain syndrome. Pain 1999;80:95–101.

42  Juottonen K, Gockel M, Silen T, Hurri H, Hari R, Forss N: Altered central sensorimotor processing in patients with complex regional pain syndrome. Pain 2002;98:315–323.

43  Schattschneider J, Wenzelburger GD, Baron R: Kinematic analysis of the upper extremity in CRPS; in Harden RN, Baron R, Janig W (eds): Complex Regional Pain Syndrome. Progr Pain Res Manage. Seattle, IASP Press, 2001, vol 22, pp 119–128.

44  Janig W, Baron R: Complex regional pain syndrome is a disease of the central nervous system. Clin Auton Res 2002;12:150–164.

45  Koltzenburg M, Wall PD, McMahon SB: Does the right side know what the left side is doing? Trends Neurosci 1999;22:122–127.

46  Haythornthwaite JA, Benrud-Larson LM: Psychological aspects of neuropathic pain. Clin J Pain 2000;16:S100–S105.

47  Oerlemans HM, Oostendorp RA, de Boo T, Goris RJ: Pain and reduced mobility in complex regional pain syndrome I: Outcome of a prospective randomised controlled clinical trial of adjuvant physical therapy versus occupational therapy. Pain 1999;83:77–83.

48  Raja SN, Grabow TS: Complex regional pain syndrome I (reflex sympathetic dystrophy). Anesthesiology 2002;96:1254–1260.

Theodore S. Grabow, MD
Assistant Professor of Anesthesiology/CCM
The Johns Hopkins Hospital – Osler 292
600 N. Wolfe St., Baltimore, MD 21287 (USA)
Tel. +1 410 955 1822, Fax +1 410 614 2019, E-Mail tgrabow@jhmi.edu

Clark MR, Treisman GJ (eds): Pain and Depression. An Interdisciplinary Patient-Centered
Approach. Adv Psychosom Med. Basel, Karger, 2004, vol 25, pp 102–122

·····················

# Can We Prevent a Second 'Gulf War Syndrome'? Population-Based Healthcare for Chronic Idiopathic Pain and Fatigue after War[1]

*Charles C. Engel*[a,b], *Ambereen Jaffer*[b], *Joyce Adkins*[b], *James R. Riddle*[c],
*Roger Gibson*[d]

[a]Department of Psychiatry, School of Medicine, Uniformed Services University,
Bethesda, Md., [b]Deployment Health Clinical Center, Walter Reed Army Medical
Center, Washington, D.C., and [c]Armed Forces Epidemiologic Board and [d]Office of
the Assistant Secretary of Defense for Health Affairs, Falls Church, Va., USA

---

### Abstract

In the 1991 Gulf War less than 150 of nearly 700,000 deployed US troops were killed
in action. Today, however, over 1 in 7 US veterans of the war has sought federal healthcare
for related-health concerns, and fully 17% of UK Gulf War veterans describe themselves as
suffering from the 'Gulf War syndrome', a set of poorly defined and heterogeneous ailments
consisting mainly of chronic pain, fatigue, depression and other symptoms. Even though
over 250 million dollars of federally funded medical research has failed to identify a unique
syndrome, the debate regarding potential causes continues and has included oil well smoke,
contagious infections, exposure to chemical and biological warfare agents, and posttraumatic
stress disorder. Historical analyses completed since the Gulf War have found that postwar
syndromes consisting of chronic pain, fatigue, depression and other symptoms have occurred
after every war in the 20th century. These syndromes have gone by a variety of names such
as Da Costa's syndrome, irritable heart, shell shock, neurocirculatory asthenia, and battle
fatigue. Though the direct causes of these syndromes are typically elusive, it is clear that war
sets in motion an undeniable cycle of physical, emotional, and fiscal consequences for war
veterans and for society. These findings lead to important healthcare questions. Is there a way to
prevent or mitigate subsequent postwar symptoms and associated depression and disability? We

[1]The views expressed in this article are those of the authors and do not necessarily
represent the official policy or position of the Uniformed Services University of the Health
Sciences, Walter Reed Army Medical Center, Department of the Army, Department of Defense,
or the US Government.

argue that while idiopathic symptoms are certain to occur following any war, a population-based approach to postwar healthcare can mitigate the impact of postwar syndromes and foster societal, military, and veteran trust. This article delineates the model, describes its epidemiological foundations, and details examples of how it is being adopted and improved as part of the system of care for US military personnel, war veterans and families. A scientific test of the model's overall effectiveness is difficult, yet healthcare systems for combatants and their families are already being put to pragmatic tests as troops return from war in Iraq and Afghanistan and from other military challenges.

## Introduction

In 1991, the United States military moved nearly 700,000 personnel to the Gulf War theater of operations over a 6-month period and with the help of a multinational coalition force rapidly extricated Iraq from Kuwait. In the process, only 147 US troops were killed in action, and the rates of disease and nonbattle injuries among these troops were similarly low [1]. Today, however, over 1 in 7 US veterans of the war has sought government-sponsored healthcare for related health concerns [2]. Fully 17% of UK Gulf War veterans describe themselves as suffering from the 'Gulf War syndrome' [3], a set of poorly defined and heterogeneous ailments consisting mainly of chronic pain, fatigue, depression and other idiopathic symptoms. Nearly 30% of US Gulf War veterans have sought service-connected disability benefits and nearly 87% of processed claims have resulted in benefits, including some 3,200 of the more than 11,000 claims for a heterogeneous set of 'undiagnosed illnesses' [4] that usually involve some combination of chronic pain, fatigue, and depression.

More than 250 million dollars spent on US government-funded medical research has failed to identify any consistent elevations in disease-related mortality or hospitalization rates among these veterans [5]. Epidemiological studies have consistently shown an excess of nearly every reportable symptom among Gulf War veterans compared to nondeployed military personnel from the Gulf War era [6], but these symptoms have failed to lead investigators to the identification of any single responsible disease or illness. The inconclusive debate regarding potential causes of pain, depression, and other idiopathic symptoms among the veterans has been fierce and confusing while implicating widely divergent factors from oil well smoke, potentially contagious infections and chemical and biological warfare agents to major depression, posttraumatic stress disorder and somatization [7, 8].

The Gulf War syndrome debate has prompted medical historians to rediscover an extensive international literature on poorly understood postwar symptom syndromes. These syndromes have followed virtually every war dating back at least as far as the Crimean War of the 1850s and have gone by a variety of different names (e.g., Da Costa's syndrome, soldier's heart, shell shock, neurocirculatory asthenia, battle fatigue) [9]. In each case, the causes of these postwar syndromes have remained elusive, but polarized etiological debates focused on competing psychological vulnerability versus biomedical disease explanations. In these postwar debates, various stakeholder groups have frequently taken up predictable and at times self-interested positions, waging well-publicized battles over the legitimacy of putative exposures and potentially related postwar symptom syndromes [8].

These etiological contests and their associated scientific, political, legal, and media debates may have unintended public health consequences including social divisions, unwarranted community health worries, and elevated mistrust between conflict veterans and the healthcare systems and individual providers that are charged with meeting their postwar health needs. These debates and the distress resulting from them may also alter potentially important health behaviors such as care-seeking, compliance with medical advice, and alcohol and tobacco use, and these behaviors can compound usual medical and psychosocial sources of symptoms and disability. In these and other ways, each war sets into motion an expanding legacy of chronic physical, emotional, and fiscal consequences that ultimately affect not only veterans but the larger society as well.

Prevailing disease management approaches to prevention and healthcare delivery do not adequately address the symptoms and disability that occur among war veterans in the weeks, months, and years following wartime environmental and psychosocial exposures. There is, therefore, a critical need for innovative and comprehensive models that can better address postwar pain, fatigue, depression, and other idiopathic symptoms. This need is particularly poignant given the recent return of US and UK military forces to Iraq and the mission to remain there during the postwar period.

Can we prevent what may become the latest in the long line of postwar syndromes or are we destined for a second version of the 'Gulf War syndrome'? Scientifically, the question remains unanswered. Our objectives in this article are to: (1) elaborate a model of postwar healthcare that targets the impact of postwar pain, fatigue, depression, and other idiopathic symptoms on relevant individuals and populations, (2) describe examples of US attempts to develop and adopt the model in the years since the 1991 Gulf War, and (3) discuss future public health and health services research initiatives necessary to sustain, further develop, and improve implementation efforts.

**Table 1.** Common predisposing, precipitating, and perpetuating factors that determine the natural history of chronic idiopathic pain, fatigue, and associated disability [22]

| Predisposing factors | Precipitating factors | Perpetuating factors |
|---|---|---|
| (1) Heredity<br>(2) Early life adversity<br>(3) Chronic illness<br>(4) Chronic distress or mental illness | (1) Biological stressors<br>(2) Acute physical illness<br>(3) Psychosocial stressors<br>(4) Acute psychiatric disorders<br>(5) Epidemic health concerns | (1) Harmful illness beliefs<br>(2) Labeling effects<br>(3) Misinformation<br>(4) Workplace and compensation factors<br>(5) Social support factors<br>(6) Physical inactivity<br>(7) Chronic illness<br>(8) Poorly integrated care |

## Disease, Symptoms, and Disability in Populations and in Clinical Practice

What can we learn from the empirical and theoretical literature on chronic idiopathic pain, fatigue, depression, and related disability that can help us develop a model of population-based healthcare for postwar symptoms? These chronic symptoms and many other idiopathic symptoms and syndromes are a significant problem in general. Conservative estimates suggest that 25–30% of people's symptoms are idiopathic [10]. Primary care physicians identify a medical explanation for symptoms in less than 1 of 7 patients in whom a medical explanation is not apparent during the initial visit and associated evaluation [11]. Chronic pain, fatigue and other idiopathic symptoms increase healthcare use but usual invasive medical approaches applied to these symptoms lead more often to iatrogenic harm, patient dissatisfaction, and provider frustration than medical benefit or patient reassurance [12, 13]. Chronic symptoms, idiopathic or not, contribute substantially to patient levels of disability [14, 15].

Chronic pain, fatigue, and other idiopathic symptoms are a source of substantial population morbidity. These symptoms and associated disability often lead to and are produced by distress, worry, anxiety, and depression [16–19]. These symptoms vary widely in severity from single symptoms that are mild and transient to multiple symptoms that are chronic, and disabling [20]. Clinical outcomes related to chronic pain, fatigue and other idiopathic symptoms are strongly correlated with biopsychosocial influences that may be characterized as predisposing, precipitating, and perpetuating factors (see table 1) [21, 22]. Cognitive factors (e.g., community or individual beliefs regarding the nature and health impact of war-related environmental and psychological exposures), behavioral factors (e.g., patterns of healthcare use), and health service experience (e.g., iatrogenic harm and differing provider and patient explanations for symptoms) may hasten the onset and perpetuate the course of these symptoms and related disability [22].

Similarly, clinical approaches can either mitigate chronic pain, fatigue and other idiopathic symptoms, or they can worsen and perpetuate them. Research has identified evidence-based treatments for chronic pain, fatigue and associated disability [23, 24]. Alternatively, differing provider and patient explanations for these symptoms and disability contribute to the frustration and dissatisfaction with care consistently observed in empirical studies [25–27]. If a healthcare visit for chronic pain or fatigue occurs in the context of community debate over cause of or blame for symptoms and disability, the provider-patient relationship may be more likely than usual to become strained, outwardly adversarial, or result in mutual rejection [28, 29]. At other times, the provider may unwittingly overrespond to these symptoms, embarking on an overly aggressive quest for causes, an approach that often leads to iatrogenic harm rather than symptom relief [12]. A bad healthcare encounter may foster provider-patient differences, disagreements, and mistrust over symptoms that tend to mirror overarching community debates [28]. Alternatively, collaborative negotiation of differing physician-patient perceptions of illness and development of a mutually acceptable model of illness may lead to increased patient satisfaction and decreased physical health concern [30].

The next part of this paper attempts to parlay this current understanding of chronic pain, fatigue and other idiopathic symptoms and into an effective model of postwar or postdisaster population-based healthcare.

## The Conceptual Basis of Population-Based Care

The goal of population-based healthcare is to achieve maximum efficiency and effectiveness through an optimized mix of population-level and individual-level interventions. These levels of care are linked together through primary care using a public health approach involving passive and active health surveillance.

Population-level care employs interventions that affect whole populations. Examples include public service announcements (e.g., antismoking campaigns) or changes in laws or policies (e.g., speed limit reduction) [31]. Individual-level care, in contrast, uses interventions that target specific patient groups defined by a common illness or service need. Both of these approaches have strengths and weaknesses. Exposure of an entire community to an intervention as occurs in population-level care can lead to a large community benefit even though the average benefit per individual is small. However, a population-level intervention must be exceedingly safe and relatively inexpensive, because everyone in the population is exposed to it, including many who would have remained healthy even without it. In contrast, individual-level intervention allows the use of higher risk and more costly interventions because the returns when used only in highly ill individuals may be great. A major drawback of individual-level intervention is that illnesses usually occur along a continuum of severity and risk. Many with relatively minor symptoms or needs necessarily go undiagnosed and untreated. Those symptoms and needs sum across a population, the result being that individual-level interventions address only a small proportion of the full magnitude of a health problem. Efforts to achieve and maintain an optimal mix of population- and individual-level interventions are the major features of population-based healthcare.

Population-based care relies on organized clinical (i.e., individual-level) services linked through primary care to a program of preclinical and population-level prevention. For this to work efficiently, community subgroups with elevated risk or with current symptoms and disability must be identified, and a mechanism to track health outcomes and help match key subgroups to specific interventions must be devised [32].

Within the population, only a small proportion of incident pain or fatigue become chronic, but individuals with these chronic symptoms are seen more frequently in healthcare settings than are individuals with transient symptoms [22]. This spectrum of chronicity, severity, and healthcare use results in a healthcare system gradient: individuals from general population samples report the fewest symptoms and least severe illness on average, those from specialty care samples report the most, and individuals from primary care samples report intermediate levels [33]. This distribution of pain, fatigue, and other idiopathic symptoms across various levels of care has implications for when, where, and how to intervene (e.g., preclinical, primary care, or tertiary care) to reduce the overall community burden of idiopathic postwar pain and fatigue. Incidence reduction (preventing first onset of postwar symptoms) generally relies on population-level interventions applied before postwar symptoms and disability occur (i.e., before healthcare is sought for them).

Efforts to reduce duration and prevent future episodes of postwar symptoms and disability are best achieved in the primary care setting because this tends to be where care is first sought. Additional attempts to reduce morbidity associated with chronic postwar symptoms and disability (e.g., psychosocial distress, psychiatric disorders, and decrements in occupational functioning) may be best initiated in primary care settings with on-site assistance from selected specialists (i.e., 'collaborative primary care'). Intensive specialty care programs for postwar symptoms and disability are then used for those who are

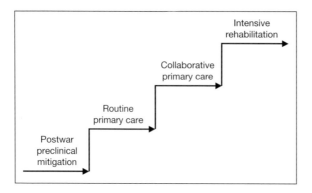

*Fig. 1.* Schematic of population-based healthcare for chronic idiopathic postwar pain, fatigue, and associated disability.

refractory to interventions at these other levels and emphasize rehabilitative efforts to increase functioning and reduce iatrogenic harm due to overaggressive or invasive diagnostic and therapeutic strategies. Figure 1 and table 2 offer a schematic and summary description, respectively, of each level of care in our model. The next section of the paper presents these levels of care in greater detail.

## Levels of Care for Chronic Postwar Pain and Fatigue

### Preclinical Prevention

Upon return from war, efforts to mitigate chronic symptoms and related disability can focus on risk groups based on the level of psychosocial, medical, and geographic proximity to traumatic events or environmental exposures (see table 3). For example, the military medical system response to the September 11 Pentagon attack used several measures of proximity to estimate risk [34]. Decreasing levels of geographic proximity included the attacked 'wedge' of the Pentagon, the rest of the Pentagon, and the National Capital Region. Exposures of concern included the physically injured, those attending to the injured or killed, those otherwise physically exposed (e.g., felt the blast, inhaled smoke, reported other environmental exposures), and those who observed people getting injured. Levels of emotional proximity included family, friends, colleagues, and subordinates of those injured or killed, of those in the damaged wedge, and of those working elsewhere in the Pentagon.

Several commonly used postwar preventive psychosocial interventions are in need of systematic evaluation. Chaos, loss of control, multiple health fears,

**Table 2.** Overview of a stepped approach to population-based healthcare for postwar idiopathic pain and fatigue

| Step | Emphasis | Setting | Goal | General approach | Information systems |
|------|----------|---------|------|------------------|---------------------|
| 1 | Postwar symptom prevention | Preclinical | Incidence and prevalence reduction | General prevention efforts based on exposures and proximity | Identify precipitating events |
| 2 | Routine primary care symptom mitigation | Primary care | Identification and prevalence reduction | Primary care provider delivers diagnostic services, low intensity treatments, and psychosocial support | Identify symptoms and concerns |
| 3 | Collaborative primary care symptom reduction and disability prevention | Primary care | Prevalence reduction | Interdisciplinary practice team intensifies care in coordination with primary care provider | Identify persistent symptoms or concerns |
| 4 | Intensive rehabilitative reduction of symptom duration and disability severity | Specialty care | Morbidity reduction | Specialized multidisciplinary and multifaceted rehabilitative programs | Identify persistent symptoms or concerns combined with disability |

**Table 3.** Preclinical modalities used to prevent chronic idiopathic postwar pain and fatigue

Workplace screening
Workplace education and support networks
Informal ('lay') debriefings
Family education and support networks

and chronic pain, fatigue and other idiopathic symptoms are common after catastrophic events including war. Workplace educational approaches teach workers about health risks and psychosocial responses to war. Community and workplace leaders often facilitate an early return to usual work routines and other roles in an effort to maximize postattack productivity. Town hall-style meetings in which leaders address community concerns provide forums for information dissemination and feedback to leaders from members of the community. Telephone 'hot lines' also afford personalized contact to people with health-related questions or concerns or who desire clinical care.

Some advocate wide-scale preclinical psychological debriefings. However, randomized controlled trials of psychological debriefings have shown no efficacy and even potential for harm [35]. Perhaps this is not surprising given that the majority of individuals do well after a traumatic experience and can therefore only experience potential adverse effects (e.g., medicalization of traumatic distress, exaggerated expectation of a poor outcome). In addition wide-scale preclinical debriefings are seldom feasible to perform with appropriate quality control procedures. Workplace liability concerns and overwhelming community desires to help victims often fuel preclinical debriefings, but scarce community resources may be better directed toward targeted clinical efforts to recognize and intervene early for adverse trauma-related outcomes including chronic pain, fatigue and other idiopathic symptoms.

Population-based preclinical screening is another commonly considered postwar strategy. Screening involves identification of individuals in need of clinical management (individual-level intervention delivered in a healthcare setting). Surveillance, by comparison, is the use of active and passive health measurement strategies to characterize the health of a community and its subgroups. It is often assumed that screening is harmless, but population-based preclinical screening has the potential to unnecessarily medicalize psychosocial concerns, and there are often significant problems with false-negative and false-positive findings. Particularly in military and other occupational settings, forced screening has the paradoxical potential to stigmatize the exact problems one is seeking to identify for the purpose of providing care. Instead, screening for postwar symptoms and disability in the privacy of the primary care setting, clinical tracking of associated outcomes, and intensification of treatment for those with identified needs is the approach we currently recommend [22].

### Routine Primary Care Mitigation of Postwar Symptoms

Chronic postwar pain and fatigue, among other idiopathic symptoms, should be expected even after relatively successful implementation of preclinical prevention programs, because clearly effective preclinical strategies are lacking. Data from the general population suggest that virtually all individuals with chronic postwar pain and fatigue will see a primary care provider over the course of a year [33]. Therefore, a key population-based healthcare response following war is early primary care recognition of these and other idiopathic postwar symptoms (see table 4). Once identified, providers can administer modest individual-level interventions to mitigate the impact of the precipitating event and reduce the potential for perpetuating factors to prolong the symptoms and their related disability. The focus on intensifying treatment for those

**Table 4.** Modalities for routine primary care mitigation of chronic idiopathic postwar pain and fatigue

| |
|---|
| Patient screening for symptoms and distress |
| Patient education regarding chronic pain and fatigue, depression, and distress |
| Management of depression |
| Clinician reminders |
| Clinician feedback regarding patient outcomes |
| Systematic consultation based on complications, nonresponse/persistence |

seeking care helps avoid stigma that may be introduced by preclinical screening and referral.

Because the symptoms linked to disability in the primary care setting are often idiopathic [14], a patient-centered approach is most comprehensive. An appropriate approach involves initial diagnostics directed toward clinical suspicions with watchful waiting to ensue if the evaluation is negative. In parallel, provider and patient collaboratively negotiate the nature, probable cause, and treatment focus. Assessment of depressive and anxiety disorders and, when necessary, introduction of related treatment options should occur early and openly. Providers often fail to communicate the degree of diagnostic uncertainty inherent in clinical practice, and they often equate 'absence of an explanation' to 'psychological explanation', alienating many patients in the process.

Instead, given the expected relationship between war, distress, mental illness, idiopathic symptoms, and disability, the possibility of future mental health consultation should be destigmatized by describing it early to patients as 'a routine part of caring for patients distressed by disabling postwar pain and fatigue'. That way patients later referred to psychiatry may be less likely to feel their primary care provider is rejecting them or contesting the validity of their symptoms. Primary care provider attempts to understand a patient's views and expectations regarding chronic postwar pain and fatigue may result in short-term improvements in patient satisfaction and provider-perceived difficulty of the encounter [36], and these efforts may enhance patient-provider trust more than blanket provider reassurances. Some 'no nonsense' providers often prefer to directly confront illness worry, but these confrontations often offend patients and disrupt continuity of care. Efforts to offer explanations, answer questions, display empathy, and define problems the patient considers relevant are advised and may be aided with timely and customized literature on common postwar concerns, symptoms, and illnesses.

The clinical decision to invoke the next level of care for postwar symptoms and disability, collaborative primary care, hinges on the persistence of symptoms

**Table 5.** Modalities for collaborative primary care reduction of chronic idiopathic postwar pain and fatigue

---

Interdisciplinary practice team with primary care provider
  integration
Clinical risk communication (up-to-date health risk
  information for clinicians and patients)
Patient education regarding symptoms and disability
Physical and psychosocial reactivation efforts
Negotiated goal setting
Collaborative problem solving

---

and associated disability, whether the patient adheres to self-care and follow-up, and whether complicating medical problems exist.

### Collaborative Primary Care Symptom Reduction and Disability Prevention

As chronic postwar pain, fatigue, and other idiopathic symptoms become more chronic and disabling for both patient and primary care provider, many setting-specific barriers to symptom management become problematic (e.g., lack of provider time). There comes a point at which postwar symptoms and disability either improve with primary care management or they persist such that the patient requires intensified individual-level approaches. Once idiopathic pain, fatigue, and disability persist beyond about 3–6 months, routine primary care management typically requires supplementation by a specialist operating from within the primary care setting, described here as 'collaborative primary care'.

A summary of collaborative primary care approaches may be found in table 5. An interdisciplinary practice team located in primary care is central [37]. Involvement of the practice team in a parallel process of multifaceted care delivered in the primary care setting provides options for physicians when options are otherwise few and provider-patient tensions may be developing. In the postwar context, this parallel, interdigitated process of care also affords patients with more intensive opportunities to communicate concerns about possible 'toxic' environmental hazards encountered during the war, to engage all available social supports, and to get assistance initiating physical and psychological activation strategies aimed at distress and disability reduction. Using the primary care clinic to deliver psychosocial and behavioral treatments minimizes potential stigma sometimes associated with these measures and it keeps care simple for patients. This may improve rates of follow-up and foster continued involvement of primary care providers, making the primary care provider more approachable and keeping provider-patient communication channels open.

Research on successful standardized consultation for idiopathic symptoms in general suggests useful practice team responsibilities and is covered elsewhere in detail [38, 39]. By and large, the practice team should ensure that patients with chronic postwar pain, fatigue and associated disability have a single primary care physician that coordinates care, sees them regularly, and applies invasive diagnostic testing and potentially disabling pharmacotherapies sparingly. The practice team helps the primary care physician to foster active coping including intensive education and modest physical activity as appropriate, to coordinate interdisciplinary treatment planning meetings, and to monitor for the need to refer to more intensive levels of care. Practice team interventions are best administered in a stepped fashion so that simple approaches are offered first and more intensive approaches are offered if these fail or if the illness trajectory suggests intensive approaches are needed.

Common elements of collaborative primary care include screening, on-site mental health consultation, cognitive-behavioral and problem-solving therapies aimed at medication adherence, depression, idiopathic symptoms and disability, physical activation and relapse prevention, videotapes, pamphlets and other education materials on self-care, structured follow-up that relies on multiple methods (visits, telephone, email, or web-internet), and longitudinal case management [for an example, see 40]. Practice teams can also enhance so-called 'risk communication', that is communications regarding potential health risks (often regarding toxic environmental hazards) that occur in a 'low-trust, high-concern' context such as the aftermath of war. In the primary care setting, if a patient harbors conspiracy fantasies or other harmful beliefs, the practice team can listen to patient concerns and beliefs, help patients test or verify them, and implement strategies when appropriate that prevent these beliefs from interfering with the patient's own care.

*Intensive Rehabilitative Care to Reduce Symptom Duration and Disability Severity*

Intensive rehabilitative care approaches are summarized in table 6. Model programs for chronic postwar pain, fatigue and associated idiopathic symptoms and disability are usually multifaceted and multidisciplinary, occur in specialized (i.e., nonprimary care) settings, and involve either a 3- to 4-week inpatient or intensive outpatient program or a 10- to 15-week program of weekly or biweekly individual or group visits [23, 41]. Medical and psychosocial approaches are combined with a structured and supervised physical activation plan. These programs view disability as a behavior amenable to modification, regardless of medical etiology.

Commonly employed cognitive-behavioral approaches to chronic idiopathic pain, fatigue, and disability help patients test their beliefs regarding cause,

***Table 6.*** Characteristics of intensive rehabilitation programs for reducing duration and disability associated with chronic idiopathic postwar pain and fatigue

---

3-week inpatient or 10- to 15-week outpatient
Structured and intensive
Multimodal
Physical and psychological reactivation
Graduated return to work
Planned practice team follow-up

---

prognosis, and treatment and identify those that are delaying progress rather than fostering improved function. Empirical trials have shown the benefits of cognitive behavioral therapy for a range of idiopathic symptom syndromes and associated disability [23, 42–45].

Physical activation is another clinical strategy that has been shown to have a number of positive effects on health and well-being across many health conditions, and efforts to bolster physical activation and functioning are common in multifaceted programs for chronic symptoms and disability [46–49]. Evidence favors supervised, graduated, and early return to work for improving role functioning for people with chronic symptoms and disability. For example, studies of patients with low back pain suggest that a return to modified work can be successful [50], while work restrictions diminish the likelihood of return to work and do not reduce absenteeism or back pain recurrences [51].

## Health Information Systems for Postwar Healthcare

The backbone for population-based care is carefully designed information systems [32]. Information systems are computer-automated systems designed to capture data that can be used to inform clinicians regarding patient status, assist clinicians and medical executives interested in monitoring and improving the quality of care, and guide policy makers attempting to assess population needs and determining appropriate staffing levels (see table 7). Information systems for facilitating care of chronic postwar pain, fatigue and disability depends on essentially three components: (1) health information systems – 'passive' computer-automated health surveillance systems that capture data that is mainly input by providers (e.g., prescriptions, diagnoses, referrals) during routine healthcare processes; (2) health monitoring systems – 'active' health surveillance systems capture patient-reported data using brief surveys and similar methods, and (3) expert computer systems – automated data processing that results in useful reports that identify high-risk patients and patient groups and

**Table 7.** Information tools for informing providers and community leaders regarding individual and community health responses to war

| |
| --- |
| Health information systems: passive computer-automated health surveillance |
| Health monitoring systems: active survey-based health surveillance |
| Expert computer systems: automated reporting to identify high-risk groups |

provide feedback for clinicians and policy makers regarding indicators of healthcare quality.

The health information system records prioritized medical problem lists and measures of healthcare use (e.g., outpatient, inpatient, and pharmacy services and various procedures), healthcare costs, presenting symptoms, primary care physician, usual place of care, patient contact information, and disease-specific data for developing registries [52]. These data, combined with data from active health monitoring approaches (e.g., patient-reported symptoms and disability), may be used to identify high-, intermediate-, and low-risk groups for intervention and tracking.

Expert computer systems process raw surveillance data into usable tools for community leaders and healthcare providers. Expert system tools aid clinical management, patient follow-up, treatment, and policy decisions. Examples of expert computer system tools include registries, reports, reminders, clinical indicators, feedback systems, guideline recommendations, and identification of appropriate patient education materials or outcome monitoring scales.

In summary, postwar preclinical, primary care, collaborative primary care, and intensive rehabilitation strategies for postwar pain, fatigue, and other idiopathic symptoms require longitudinal assessments and tracking to remain linked to one another and to facilitate population-based approaches to prevention and care. An information system comprised of health information systems, health monitoring systems, and expert computer systems is advocated for achieving these aims and bringing disparate levels of and approaches to care into communication with one another.

### Preventing Postwar Syndromes – Implementing the Strategy

What evidence exists that the population-based healthcare approach we describe is feasible or effective? Admittedly, efforts are in an early stage, but a series of research, policy, and practice initiatives focused within the US

Department of Defense (DoD) offer examples to suggest the model is feasible and that some elements are effective. In addition, these initiatives suggest the model may offer a roadmap for improving community health system response to events of homeland security and public health significance [53]. We highlight three illustrative advances occurring with the DoD: (1) development of a postwar health services research agenda and expertise, (2) implementation of primary care practice guidelines on postdeployment healthcare delivery, and (3) exploration of novel guideline implementation strategies following the terrorist attacks of September 11, 2001. The following discussion offers descriptions of these advances.

### Postwar Health Services Research Agenda and Expertise

In the early 1990s concerns over a possible Gulf War syndrome helped crystallize understanding that the DoD needed an ongoing postwar health services research agenda and a specific cadre of scientific and clinical expertise. In response to these concerns, the department initiated the Comprehensive Clinical Evaluation Program (CCEP) in 1994. The CCEP functioned as an extensive clinical diagnostic program for Gulf War veterans as well as a clinical registry to facilitate research into emerging questions regarding toxic war exposures and potentially related chronic postwar pain, fatigue, and other idiopathic symptoms [54]. The Department of Veterans Affairs (VA) had recently implemented the Persian Gulf Veterans' Registry [55] for similar purposes.

These programs, imperfect as they were, led to lessons regarding postwar healthcare delivery [55, 56], completion of research [22, 55, 57–59], and feedback from veterans [56]. In 1999 the DoD established the Deployment Health Clinical Center with the mission of improving postdeployment healthcare using clinical, health services research, and educational approaches.

An intensive rehabilitative program for Gulf War veterans with persistent or treatment refractory symptoms was developed for the CCEP [60]. The program, still in existence, employs chronic disease management, graded physical activation, and cognitive-behavioral approaches as key therapeutic elements. The program has now treated veterans of other conflicts with similar symptoms and military service-related health concerns to those of Gulf War veterans.

Two of these essential rehabilitative elements, graded physical activation and cognitive-behavioral therapy, were evaluated in a randomized controlled trial carried out at eighteen VA and two DoD sites. Exercise and cognitive behavioral therapy were chosen for study because of their demonstrated efficacy in controlled trials of patients with similar idiopathic symptom syndromes such as fibromyalgia and chronic fatigue syndrome [23, 42, 46, 47, 61]. The VA/DoD trial, described in greater detail elsewhere [62], evaluated 1-year treatment outcomes for nearly 1,100 Gulf War veterans with chronic idiopathic postwar pain, fatigue, and associated disability. The Centers for Disease Control and Prevention (CDC) developed the case definition employed in the trial, called 'chronic multisymptom illness', using statistical and clinical methods [63]. In a two-by-two factoral research design, veterans were randomized to one of four treatment arms that delivered 12 weeks of either physical activation, group cognitive behavioral therapy, or both versus usual postwar symptomatic care. Results were similar to those found in our pilot studies [64], revealing modest improvements in symptoms of fatigue and cognitive impairment and in mental health functioning with both graded activity and with cognitive-behavioral therapy [62]. While the approach is not curative, it offered some symptom relief and improved quality of life for many veterans with chronic postwar pain, fatigue, and disability.

The combined strategy of postwar registries, intensive postwar rehabilitative programs, and a center of postwar healthcare delivery and research expertise emerged from the health concerns of 1991 Gulf War veterans and represents advances in postwar military healthcare.

*Primary Care Practice Guidelines on Postdeployment Healthcare Delivery*

In evaluating the adequacy of the VA and DoD diagnostic programs for Gulf War veterans, healthcare scientists representing the Institute of Medicine concluded that a systematic quality improvement program was needed for these postwar healthcare programs. The panel recommended clinical practice guidelines as one important early step in achieving that objective [55]. Consequently, beginning in 1999, a collaboration with nearly fifty clinicians, scientists, and health policy experts from the federal sector and academic medicine developed a clinical practice guideline for assessing, evaluating, and treating returning service members with deployment-related health concerns. This guideline, called the Department of Defense and Veterans Health Administration Clinical Practice Guideline for Post-Deployment Evaluation and Management (PDH-CPG; see http://www.pdhealth.mil/clinicians/PDHEM/ToolKit/view/2/guideline_ver1.2.doc), underwent piloting in 2001 at selected medical facilities from high deployment sites in the Army, Air Force, Navy, and Marine Corps with final implementation in early 2002 [65]. Complementary practice guidelines were developed for use among those patients identified in postwar assessments with chronic idiopathic pain and fatigue or with major depressive disorder (see http://www.oqp.med.va.gov/cpg/cpg.htm). All of these practice guidelines employed a process of evidence-based guideline development and implementation organized with the assistance of RAND Corporation investigators [66].

The main goal of PDH-CPG is to facilitate, support, and improve the care provided for recently deployed veterans with postwar or postdeployment health concerns, and the guideline has already spawned new health services research and clinical quality improvement efforts. Features of PDH-CPG include an emphasis on primary care, primary care screening for deployment or war-related health concerns, and centralized web-based risk communication and clinician implementation support (see PDHealth.mil at http://www.pdhealth.mil). PDH-CPG offers clinical evaluation and follow-up guidance, a clinical framework for communicating effectively about military-related health risks, and other supporting clinical and patient education tools. Several indicators ('metrics') are used to help track guideline implementation.

Screening for health concerns is facilitated using a 'military-unique vital sign'. Evidence suggests that this vital sign effectively identifies patients with idiopathic physical symptoms, depression, general psychosocial distress, and low satisfaction with care [67]. PDH-CPG prescribes that all DoD beneficiaries visiting primary care clinics get routinely asked, 'Is your visit today for a deployment-related health concern?' The answer is recorded as yes, no, or maybe. Affirmative responses prompt care in accordance with the guideline. To facilitate development of population-based registries of individuals with deployment-related health concerns, visits that the patient reports are due to a deployment-related health concern are coded using an ICD-9-CM V-code (v70.5_ _6).

Patients with health concerns are prescribed extra or extended visits to accommodate discussions of these concerns. Guidance to clinicians on how to facilitate communication around these concerns is offered for four types of patients: those without deployment health concerns, those with concerns who are otherwise asymptomatic, those with concerns and a diagnosable disease, and those with concerns and idiopathic symptoms (i.e., the postwar syndrome patient).

*Guideline Implementation following the September 11*
*Pentagon Attack*
Programmatic efforts to provide health services for individuals affected by the September 11 Pentagon attack help illustrate how recent postwar healthcare initiatives may also lead to advances in healthcare system response following an event with homeland security implications. The Army Medical Department initiated 'Operation Solace' in the greater Washington, D.C. area following the Pentagon attack to ensure that individuals with related health concerns received appropriate medical assistance. Piloting of PDH-CPG was nearly complete, and efforts to implement it were undertaken in area primary care portals. Primary care patients were asked a modified version of the military-unique vital sign to ascertain if a visit was due to deployment, bioterrorism, or attack-related health concerns. Each implementing clinic used an 'Operation Solace care manager'. The care manager's task was to help clinics to integrate guideline practices into their process of care. When a patient indicated a concern on the vital sign, the

care manager helped the patient and the primary care provider to elucidate September 11-related concerns, resolve barriers to care, improve continuity of care, and coordinate referrals and follow-up.

During a 6-month period in 2002, 100 patients that screened positive on the military-unique vital sign (less than 1% of all visits to area primary care clinics during the period) completed a survey to define the reason for the visit and other health status variables. Deployment was the most common reason for the patients' concern, followed by the attack. September 11-related health concerns constituted less than 1% of primary care visits to participating clinics, but compared to data from civilian primary care settings, the patients with concerns reported significant elevations in physical symptoms, posttraumatic distress, mental disorders, and healthcare use, and low levels of satisfaction with care [67].

Operation Solace illustrates how population-based healthcare approaches can leverage primary care settings to improve overall healthcare system responsiveness following war and other traumatic events. Future health services research needs to address whether the use of a care manager can improve the longitudinal care of patients with war or deployment-related health concerns, improve these patients' satisfaction with their healthcare, reduce high service use, and maximize health outcomes. From a population health perspective, a public military commitment to improve healthcare for those injured in the line of duty may improve institutional trust among those who must rely on it while negotiating the hazards of war.

### Conclusion

Disease management strategies will only offer solutions for a small proportion of the symptoms and disability in a community following war. The population-based healthcare model that we have described in this paper offers solutions for healthcare systems such as the DoD and VA systems as well as for communities preparing for or previously affected by terrorist attack. This model is feasible, stepped, interdisciplinary, multifaceted, and lends itself to evaluation and improvement. It optimally combines public health perspective with patient-centered care based on individual patient needs. These linkages between public health and individual patient approaches are made with carefully planned health information systems along with an emphasis on primary care.

### References

1   Writer JV, DeFraites RF, Brundage JF: Comparative mortality among US military personnel in the Persian Gulf region and worldwide during Operations Desert Shield and Desert Storm. JAMA 1996;275/2:118–121.

2   Smith TC, Smith B, Ryan MA, Gray GC, Hooper TI, Heller JM, Dalager NA, Kang HK, Gackstetter GD: Ten years and 100,000 participants later: Occupational and other factors influencing participation in US Gulf War health registries. J Occup Environ Med 2002;44:758–768.

3   Chalder T, Hotopf M, Unwin C, Hull L, Ismail K, David A, Wessely S: Prevalence of Gulf war veterans who believe they have Gulf war syndrome: Questionnaire study. BMJ 2001;323:473–476.

4   Veterans Benefits Administration. Office of Performance Analysis and Integrity. May 2002 Gulf War Veterans Information System Briefing For: National Gulf War Resource Center. Washington, Department of Veterans Affairs, 2002.

5   Military and Veterans Health Coordinating Board Research Working Group Members: Annual Report to Congress: Federally Sponsored Research on Gulf War Veterans' Illnesses for 2001. Washington, Department of Veterans Affairs, 2002.

6   Unwin C, Blatchley N, Coker W, Ferry S, Hotopf M, Hull L, Ismail K, Palmer I, David A, Wessely S: Health of UK servicemen who served in Persian Gulf War. Lancet 1999;353:169–178.

7   Riddle JR, Brown M, Smith T, Ritchie EC, Brix KA, Romano J: Chemical warfare and the Gulf War: A review of the impact on Gulf veterans' health. Mil Med 2003;168:606–613.

8   Sartin JS: Gulf War illnesses: Causes and controversies. Mayo Clin Proc 2000;75:811–819.

9   Hyams KC, Wignall FS, Roswell R: War syndromes and their evaluation: From the U.S. Civil War to the Persian Gulf War. Ann Intern Med 1996;125:398–405.

10  Kroenke K, Price RK: Symptoms in the community. Prevalence, classification, and psychiatric comorbidity. Arch Intern Med 1993;153:2474–2480.

11  Kroenke K, Mangelsdorff AD: Common symptoms in ambulatory care: Incidence, evaluation, therapy, and outcome. Am J Med 1989;86/3:262–266.

12  Kouyanou K, Pither CE, Rabe-Hesketh S, Wessely S: A comparative study of iatrogenesis, medication abuse, and psychiatric morbidity in chronic pain patients with and without medically explained symptoms. Pain 1998;76:417–426.

13  Twemlow SW, Bradshaw SLJ, Coyne L, Lerma BH: Patterns of utilization of medical care and perceptions of the relationship between doctor and patient with chronic illness including chronic fatigue syndrome. Psychol Rep 1997;80:643–658.

14  Kroenke K, Spitzer RL, Williams JB, Linzer M, Hahn SR, deGruy FV 3rd, Brody D: Physical symptoms in primary care. Predictors of psychiatric disorders and functional impairment. Arch Fam Med 1994;3:774–779.

15  Escobar JI, Golding JM, Hough RL, Karno M, Burnam MA, Wells KB: Somatization in the community: Relationship to disability and use of services. Am J Public Health 1987;77:837–840.

16  Gureje O, Simon GE, Von Korff M: A cross-national study of the course of persistent pain in primary care. Pain 2001;92/1–2:195–200.

17  Von Korff M, Simon G: The relationship between pain and depression. Br J Psychiatry Suppl 1996;30:101–108.

18  Gureje O, Von Korff M, Simon GE, Gater R: Persistent pain and well-being: A World Health Organization Study in Primary Care. JAMA 1998;280:147–151.

19  Armenian HK, Pratt LA, Gallo J, Eaton WW: Psychopathology as a predictor of disability: A population-based follow-up study in Baltimore, Maryland. Am J Epidemiol 1998;148/3:269–275.

20  Katon W, Lin E, Von Korff M, Russo J, Lipscomb P, Bush T: Somatization: A spectrum of severity. Am J Psychiatry 1991;148/1:34–40.

21  Walker EA, Unutzer J, Katon WJ: Understanding and caring for the distressed patient with multiple medically unexplained symptoms. J Am Board Fam Pract 1998;11:347–356.

22  Engel CC, Katon WJ: Population and need-based prevention of unexplained physical symptoms in the community; in Institute of Medicine, Strategies to Protect the Health of Deployed U.S. Forces: Medical Surveillance, Record Keeping, and Risk Reduction. Washington, National Press, 1999, pp 173–212.

23  Kroenke K, Swindle R: Cognitive-behavioral therapy for somatization and symptom syndromes: A critical review of controlled clinical trials. Psychosom Psychother 2000;69/4:205–215.

24  O'Malley PG, Jackson JL, Santoro J, Tomkins G, Balden E, Kroenke K: Antidepressant therapy for unexplained symptoms and symptom syndromes. J Fam Pract 1999;48:980–990.

25  Hahn SR, Thompson KS, Wills TA, Stern V, Budner NS: The difficult doctor-patient relationship: Somatization, personality and psychopathology. J Clin Epidemiol 1994;47:647–657.

26    Lin EH, Katon W, Von Korff M, Bush T, Lipscomb P, Russo J, Wagner E: Frustrating patients: Physician and patient perspectives among distressed high users of medical services. J Gen Intern Med 1991;6:241–246.

27    Walker EA, Katon WJ, Keegan D, Gardner G, Sullivan M: Predictors of physician frustration in the care of patients with rheumatological complaints. Gen Hosp Psychiatry 1997;19:315–323.

28    Engel CC, Adkins JA, Cowan DN: Caring for medically unexplained physical symptoms after toxic environmental exposures: Effects of contested causation. Environ Health Perspect 2002;110(suppl 4): 641–647.

29    Quill TE: Somatization disorder. One of medicine's blind spots. JAMA 1985;254:3075–3079.

30    Von Korff M, Gruman J, Schaefer J, Curry SJ, Wagner EH: Collaborative management of chronic illness. Ann Intern Med 1997;127:1097–1102.

31    Rose G: The Strategy of Preventive Medicine. New York, Oxford University Press, 1992.

32    Wagner EH, Austin BT, Von Korff M: Organizing care for patients with chronic illness. Milbank Q 1996;74:511–544.

33    Green LA, Fryer GEJ, Yawn BP, Lanier D, Dovey SM: The ecology of medical care revisited. N Engl J Med 2001;344:2021–2025.

34    Orman DT, Robichaux RJ, Crandell EO, Patterson VJ, Hoge CW, Engel CC, Ritchie EC, Milliken CS: Operation Solace: Overview of the mental health intervention following the September 11, 2001 Pentagon attack. Mil Med 2002;167(suppl 9):44–47.

35    Wessely S, Rose S, Bisson J: A systematic review of brief psychological interventions for the treatment of immediate trauma related symptoms and the prevention of posttraumatic stress disorder (Cochrane Review); in The Cochrane Library, Issue 2. Oxford, Software, 1998.

36    Jackson JL, Kroenke K, Chamberlin J: Effects of physician awareness of symptom-related expectations and mental disorders. A controlled trial. Arch Fam Med 1999;8/2:135–142.

37    Wagner EH: The role of patient care teams in chronic disease management. BMJ 2000;320:569–572.

38    Smith GRJ, Rost K, Kashner TM: A trial of the effect of a standardized psychiatric consultation on health outcomes and costs in somatizing patients. Arch Gen Psychiatry 1995;52/3:238–243.

39    Von Korff M, Moore JC: Stepped care for back pain: Activating approaches for primary care. Ann Intern Med 2001;134:911–917.

40    Powell P, Bentall RP, Nye FJ, Edwards RH: Randomised controlled trial of patient education to encourage graded exercise in chronic fatigue syndrome. BMJ 2001;322:387–390.

41    Flor H, Fydrich T, Turk DC: Efficacy of multidisciplinary pain treatment centers: A meta-analytic review. Pain 1992;49:221–230.

42    Price JR, Couper J: Cognitive behaviour therapy for adults with chronic fatigue syndrome. Cochrane Database Syst Rev 2000;2:CD001027.

43    Deale A, Husain K, Chalder T, Wessely S: Long-term outcome of cognitive behavior therapy versus relaxation therapy for chronic fatigue syndrome: A 5-year follow-up study. Am J Psychiatry 2001;158:2038–2042.

44    Prins JB, Bleijenberg G, Bazelmans E, Elving LD, de Boo TM, Severens JL, van der Wilt GJ, Spinhoven P, van der Meer JW: Cognitive behaviour therapy for chronic fatigue syndrome: A multi-centre randomised controlled trial. Lancet 2001;357:841–847.

45    Speckens AE, van Hemert AM, Spinhoven P, Hawton KE, Bolk JH, Rooijmans HG: Cognitive behavioural therapy for medically unexplained physical symptoms: A randomised controlled trial. BMJ 1995;311:1328–1332.

46    Wearden AJ, Morriss RK, Mullis R, Strickland PL, Pearson DJ, Appleby L, Campbell IT, Morris JA: Randomised, double-blind, placebo-controlled treatment trial of fluoxetine and graded exercise for chronic fatigue syndrome. Br J Psychiatry 1998;172:485–490.

47    Fulcher KY, White PD: Randomised controlled trial of graded exercise in patients with the chronic fatigue syndrome. BMJ 1997;314:1647–1652.

48    Frost H, Lamb SE, Klaber Moffett JA, Fairbank JC, Moser JS: A fitness programme for patients with chronic low back pain: 2-year follow-up of a randomised controlled trial. Pain 1998;75/2–3: 273–279.

49    McCain GA, Bell DA, Mai FM, Halliday PD: A controlled study of the effects of a supervised cardiovascular fitness training program on the manifestations of primary fibromyalgia. Arthritis Rheum 1988;31:1135–1141.

50   Frank JW, Brooker AS, DeMaio SE, Kerr MS, Maetzel A, Shannon HS, Sullivan TJ, Norman RW, Wells RP: Disability resulting from occupational low back pain. Part II: What do we know about secondary prevention? A review of the scientific evidence on prevention after disability begins. Spine 1996;21:2918–2929.

51   Burton AK, Erg E: Back injury and work loss. Biomechanical and psychosocial influences. Spine 1997;22:2575–2580.

52   Katon W, Von Korff M, Lin E, Unutzer J, Simon G, Walker E, Ludman E, Bush T: Population-based care of depression: Effective disease management strategies to decrease prevalence. Gen Hosp Psychiatry 1997;19/3:169–178.

53   Engel CC, Jaffer JA, Sheliga V, et al: Population-based health care: A model for restoring community health and productivity following terrorist attack; in Ursano RJ, Fullerton CS, Norwood AE (eds): Terrorism and Disaster: Individual and Community Mental Health Interventions. New York, Cambridge University Press, 2003, pp 287–307.

54   Department of Defense: Comprehensive Clinical Evaluation Program for Gulf War Veterans: CCEP Report on 18,598 Participants. Washington, Department of Defense, 1996.

55   Institute of Medicine: Adequacy of the VA Persian Gulf Registry and Uniform Case Assessment Protocol. Washington, National Academy Press, 1998.

56   Institute of Medicine: Committee on the Evaluation of the Department of Defense Comprehensive Clinical Evaluation Program. Adequacy of the Comprehensive Clinical Evaluation Program: A Focused Assessment. Washington, National Academy Press, 1997.

57   Gray GC, Hawksworth AW, Smith TC, Kang HK, Knoke JD, Gackstetter GD: Gulf War Veterans' Health Registries. Who is most likely to seek evaluation? Am J Epidemiol 1998;148: 343–349.

58   Kroenke K, Koslowe P, Roy M: Symptoms in 18,495 Persian Gulf War veterans. Latency of onset and lack of association with self-reported exposures. J Occup Environ Med 1998;40: 520–528.

59   Roy MJ, Koslowe PA, Kroenke K, Magruder C: Signs, symptoms, and ill-defined conditions in Persian Gulf War veterans: Findings from the Comprehensive Clinical Evaluation Program. Psychosom Med 1998;60:663–668.

60   Engel CC, Roy M, Kayanan D, Ursano R: Multidisciplinary treatment of persistent symptoms after Gulf War service. Mil Med 1998;163/4:202–208.

61   Richards SC, Scott DL: Prescribed exercise in people with fibromyalgia: Parallel group randomised controlled trial. BMJ 2002;325:185.

62   Donta ST, Clauw DJ, Engel CC Jr, Guarino P, Peduzzi P, Williams DA, Skinner JS, Barkhuizen A, Taylor T, Kazis LE, et al: Cognitive behavioral therapy and aerobic exercise for Gulf War veterans' illnesses: A randomized controlled trial. JAMA 2003;289:1396–1404.

63   Fukuda K, Nisenbaum R, Stewart G, Thompson WW, Robin L, Washko RM, Noah DL, Barrett DH, Randall B, Herwaldt BL, et al: Chronic multisymptom illness affecting Air Force veterans of the Gulf War. JAMA 1998;280:981–988.

64   Engel CC, Liu X, Clymer R, Miller RF, Sjoberg T, Shapiro JR: Rehabilitative care of war-related health concerns. J Occup Environ Med 2000;42:385–390.

65   Farley DO, Vernez G, Pieklik S, et al: Implementing the Post-Deployment Health Practice Guideline: Lessons from the Field Demonstration. Washington, RAND, 2002.

66   Nicholas W, Farley DO, Vaiana M, Cretin S: Putting Practice Guidelines to Work in the Department of Defense Medical System: A Guideline for Action. Santa Monica, RAND, 2001.

67   Jaffer A, Robinson R, Cowan DN, Engel CC: Somatic symptoms and psychiatric morbidity among patients seeking care after the Pentagon attack. Ann Epidemiol 2003;13:575.

Dr. C.C. Engel
Department of Psychiatry
Uniformed Services University of the Health Sciences
4301 Jones Bridge Road, Bethesda, MD 20814-4799 (USA)
Tel. +1 202 782 8064, Fax +1 202 782 3539, E-Mail cengel@usuhs.mil

Clark MR, Treisman GJ (eds): Pain and Depression. An Interdisciplinary Patient-Centered
Approach. Adv Psychosom Med. Basel, Karger, 2004, vol 25, pp 123–137

..........................

# Opioid Effectiveness, Addiction, and Depression in Chronic Pain

*Paul J. Christo, Theodore S. Grabow, Srinivasa N. Raja*

Division of Pain Medicine, Department of Anesthesiology and Critical Care
Medicine, Johns Hopkins University School of Medicine, Baltimore, Md., USA

## Abstract

Opioids are a viable treatment for chronic pain, but their use requires individualization, specified treatment goals, and patient education. Opioid responsiveness is influenced by patient-centered characteristics, including a predisposition to opioid side effects, psychological distress, and opioid use history; pain-centered characteristics, which involve the temporal pattern, rapidity of onset, severity, and type of pain; and drug-centered characteristics relating to the impact of specific types of opioids on specific patients. Thus, opioid doses should be titrated to achieve a favorable balance between analgesia and adverse effects. Opioid therapy can be enhanced through the adjunct administration of agents such as NMDA antagonists, calcium channel blockers, clonidine, and even low-dose opioid antagonists. Controversy exists over 1) the long-term use of opioids for non-cancer pain, and patients receiving opioids for long periods must be monitored carefully for signs of addictive and aberrant behavior, 2) the impact of opioid therapy on emotional depression in patients with chronic pain, and 3) whether opioid therapy causes cognitive impairment in the elderly. Our ability to determine the validity of such assertions and the exact role of opioids in the treatment of chronic pain will benefit from further study.

## Introduction

One third of the United States population will experience chronic pain. In fact, chronic pain is the most common cause of long-term disability in the United States and partially or totally disables nearly 50 million people [1]. Among the therapeutic options for treatment of chronic pain, the use of opioids remains a viable choice. Research into opioid pharmacology over the past

20 years has expanded our knowledge of the mechanism of action of opioids [2]. Many studies on patients with cancer pain have provided insight into the clinical pharmacology of opioids. Research findings support the idea that the pharmacokinetic and pharmacodynamic principles of opioids in cancer patients with pain hold true in patients with chronic, nonmalignant pain [3].

While the use of opioids for chronic cancer pain is widely accepted, the efficacy and role of opioids in the management of chronic noncancer pain has been intensely debated. Opponents argue that there is no place for opioids in the treatment of chronic benign pain and opine that narcotics are a major impediment to the successful treatment of chronic pain. This view is largely based on concerns regarding tolerance, physical dependence, addiction, and adverse affective and cognitive side effects. Supporters, in contrast, state that some types of pains, e.g., nociceptive pains, are opioid responsive, while others such as neuropathic pain might be less responsive, but not resistant. Much of this debate has occurred till recent years in the absence of randomized clinical trials. Although several recent studies have demonstrated that chronic pain, including neuropathic pain states such as postherpetic neuralgia, is responsive to opioids, these studies have followed patients for relatively short periods of 2 months or less. More careful studies of the long-term efficacy of opioids are needed to determine if tolerance to the analgesic effects of opioids limits its usefulness for long-term therapy.

## Opioid Effectiveness

The appropriate use of opioids in the management of chronic pain demands individualization [4]. That is, one opioid does not 'fit all' patients with a certain type of pain. In addition, we lack a mechanistic approach that would guide the management of chronic pain states with specific opioids. The goal in the management of a patient's pain with opioids is to achieve an optimal balance between the drug's analgesic effects and any associated adverse effects.

In 1990, Portenoy et al. [5] advanced a strategy for conceptualizing opioid effectiveness in managing patients with chronic pain. According to this strategy, the rational use of opioids should focus on achieving maximum analgesic efficacy while limiting toxicity. The success of this approach requires gradual titration of the opioid to the point at which a favorable balance between analgesia and side effects is achieved. Finding this acceptable balance between analgesia and side effects requires frequent interactions between the clinician and patient.

Several factors can influence opioid responsiveness in managing chronic pain: specifically, patient-centered characteristics, pain-centered characteristics, and drug-centered characteristics.

## Patient-Centered Characteristics

Patient-centered characteristics, such as a predisposition to opioid side effects, reduce opioid responsiveness, irrespective of pain syndrome type [5]. This predisposition may derive from higher than normal plasma levels of opioid following a single dose (pharmacokinetic) or even from an exaggerated response to modest levels of plasma opioid (pharmacodynamic). Therefore, side effects after a given dose or doses of opioid are difficult to predict but will prevent the patient from achieving a balance between analgesia and adverse effects. Further, concurrent use of other medications with additive side effects will increase the risk of intolerable opioid side effects at doses that are inadequate for analgesia.

If patients are experiencing psychological distress, they may respond less favorably to opioid therapy [6]. Among the cancer population, patients who receive psychological interventions or psychotropic medication achieve better analgesia with the same opioid and dose than do patients receiving no psychological assistance. Similarly, poor opioid responses by addicted individuals may result from affective disturbances such as depression and anxiety.

Those patients who have recently consumed large doses or escalating doses of opioids also may respond poorly to current opioid therapy. This outcome may result from disease progression among the cancer or noncancer population or may result from tolerance. It is important to remember that patients consuming high doses of an opioid at baseline will require large incremental doses to achieve analgesia.

Finally, genetic determinants may influence opioid effectiveness in patients by altering the density or proportion of opioid receptors or by changing the expression of opioid isoforms.

## Pain-Centered Characteristics

Pain-centered characteristics can influence patient responsiveness to opioids. For instance, the temporal patterns of pain exert a strong influence on opioid effectiveness [7]. If pain is of rapid onset, the opioid tends to be ineffective, perhaps due to our inability to deliver the drug fast enough. Furthermore, intermittent and severe pain often require large or quickly escalating opioid doses for pain control, but such doses often cause intolerable side effects [8].

Neuropathic pain is another pain-focused characteristic that influences opioid effectiveness. In the past, clinical observations and studies described neuropathic pain as unresponsive to opioids [9, 10]. Yet, data from clinical surveys supported a revised notion that opioids can relieve neuropathic pain

[11, 12], and controlled studies provided convincing evidence that this is true [13, 14]. Further, a randomized, placebo-controlled trial comparing the use of opioids with that of tricyclic antidepressants to treat postherpetic neuralgia found that the opioids provided superior analgesic efficacy with minimal cognitive effects [15]. In short, the evidence supports the rational use of long-term opioid treatment in patients with nonmalignant painful neuropathies and/or cancer pain. Clinically, patients with neuropathic pain probably display a reduced response to opioids compared with patients with nociceptive pain. Work by Cherny et al. [16] suggests that neuropathic pain responds to standard opioid doses, but less analgesia is achieved than for nociceptive pain, and the efficacy/side effect balance is more difficult to accomplish. Other studies add to the growing clinical concept that neuropathic mechanisms merely reduce opioid response without imparting opioid resistance [17–19].

### Drug-Centered Characteristics

Opioid responsiveness can differ according to drug-specific effects. That is, patients may experience better analgesia and fewer associated side effects with one opioid yet fail to achieve adequate analgesia with another opioid that also induces unmanageable side effects [5, 20]. The results of animal studies indicate the possibility that a relationship exists between a physiological pain mechanism (visceral vs. cutaneous) and the opioid receptor subtypes that produce analgesia. Specifically, work by Sengupta et al. [21], using experimental models of visceral pain, suggests a role for peripheral kappa receptors and not mu or delta receptors in the modulation of visceral pain. The mechanistic process may relate to the sensitivity or density of receptor subtypes or isoforms and/or to the specific binding properties of the opioids to these subtypes and isoforms.

Tolerance to the analgesic effects of opioid occurs even after a single dose of the drug in experimental animals. However, the extent to which this is a problem in the clinical use of opioids for chronic pain management is less clear. It is generally considered to be less of an issue in clinical pain states as patients can often be maintained on stable doses for prolonged periods of time [7].

*Enhancing Opioid Therapy by Adding N-Methyl-D-Aspartate*
*Antagonists, Calcium Channel Blockers, Clonidine, and Opioids*
*Plus Low-Dose Opioid Antagonists*

Insights into the process of neuroplasticity indicate that adding N-methyl-D-aspartate (NMDA) antagonists may help treat types of pain that are not optimally responsive to opioids (neuropathic pain, breakthrough pain, increased pain due to tolerance to the drug's analgesic effects) [22, 23]. The NMDA antagonists may exert more influence on the altered central processing of pain signals than on the physiological transmission of painful impulses and may produce analgesia directly or reverse tolerance. Ketamine (a noncompetitive NMDA receptor antagonist) blocks the NMDA receptor-controlled ion channel on dorsal horn neurons when a nociceptive burst releases glutamate into the synaptic cleft. Consequently, ketamine may be more effective in modifying the central hyperexcitability and 'wind-up' processes related to neuropathic as opposed to acute pain [24]. Persson et al. [25] reported a synergism between ketamine and opioids. In this study, cancer patients who lost analgesia from high-dose morphine achieved substantial analgesia while halving their morphine doses after the addition of a low dose of ketamine (110 mg/day) to the treatment regimen. Moreover, in a double-blind, crossover study, Mercandante et al. [26] reported favorable results using ketamine (0.25–0.5 mg/kg) with morphine in cancer patients suffering from uncontrolled neuropathic pain. Undesirable psychotomimetic side effects (illusions, disturbing dreams, delirium) can occur with ketamine use, however, and should be monitored and preempted using benzodiazepines or haloperidol at doses of 2–4 mg/day [27].

Animal studies suggest a critical role of NMDA receptors in modulating chronic pain states; however, the clinical efficacy of NMDA receptors in human studies has yet to be established. Methadone produces analgesia by activating mu opioid receptors, but the drug also acts as an NMDA receptor antagonist. In fact, methadone is unique among opioids and may offer greater effectiveness than the other opioids in managing neuropathic or opioid-tolerant pain [28]. Likewise, dextromethorphan (DM) acts as an NMDA antagonist, and potentiates NSAID and morphine analgesia [29]. Because DM offers a convincing safety profile as an antitussive [30] and lacks psychomimetic side effects, it may be useful in treating chronic pain conditions. However, the evidence from randomized, controlled trials on the beneficial effects of clinically available NMDA antagonists is not convincing [31, 32].

It is well known that calcium channels play a critical role in presynaptic release of neurotransmitters; therefore, blocking these channels in the context of opioid use may facilitate antinociception. Santillan et al. [33] found that the calcium channel blocker nimodipine permitted a decrease in morphine use in 16 of 23 patients but failed in 2 patients and was discontinued in 5 patients. In 1996, Roca et al. [34] reported opposing results after administering nimodipine 30 mg p.o. q8 h to cancer patients who were concurrently taking sustained-release morphine. These investigators noted no enhanced analgesia in the treatment group. Incorporating calcium channel blockers into an analgesic regimen may be limited by their hemodynamic properties.

Clonidine shows promise in enhancing opioid responsiveness in chronic pain states. Clonidine is an $\alpha_2$-adrenergic agonist and nonspecific analgesic that inhibits primary afferent transmission and substance P release from nociceptive neurons in the spinal cord [35]. The pain-relieving qualities of intraspinal clonidine have been demonstrated in patients with intractable, neuropathic cancer pain [36]. Clonidine's analgesic effect may be independent of opioid pathways [37] and may act synergistically with morphine to suppress dorsal horn neurons [38].

Growing evidence supports the role of low-dose opioid antagonists in enhancing the analgesic potency of morphine or other opioids. For instance, Levine et al. [39] demonstrated that low-dose naloxone given with pentazocine provides greater analgesia than high-dose morphine alone. These investigators studied more than 100 patients in a double-blind fashion following surgery for tooth extraction. In a double-blind study on 60 posthysterectomy patients, Gan et al. [40] infused low-dose naloxone during a 24-hour period and discovered that patient-controlled analgesia (PCA) usage of morphine decreased from 60 to 40 mg. Gan et al. concluded that naloxone increased morphine's potency, decreased tolerance, and reduced the nausea, vomiting, and pruritus associated with morphine treatment. Moreover, ultra-low-dose intravenous nalmefene (a pure mu receptor antagonist) enhanced postoperative analgesia with PCA morphine in 120 lower-abdominal surgery patients in a randomized, double-blind, placebo-controlled study [41]. The patients receiving nalmefene had a significantly decreased need for antiemetics and antipruritic medications while receiving PCA with morphine. These studies provide encouraging evidence that low-dose opioid antagonists given with opioids may enhance opioid responsiveness.

## Addiction

The role of opioids for the treatment of chronic, nonmalignant pain remains controversial, despite growing acceptance of this practice. The literature confirms the beneficial use of opioids for noncancer pain [42] but more long-term studies are needed to support the use of opioids in non-cancer pain patients.

When using opioids to manage chronic nonmalignant pain, clinicians must consider (1) whether opioids improve the patient's physical and psychological functioning and (2) the patient's potential for addiction. Pain specialists struggle to achieve a balance between improving a patient's pain through opioid use and interfering with a patient's functioning in a manner that could worsen disability or even obviate the gain in pain control. The data demonstrate that addiction is unlikely to occur due to opioid exposure in the presence of chronic pain [43], and it is not clear that the prevalence of addiction is greater in the chronic pain population than in the general population. Clinical experience in using opioids to treat cancer pain demonstrates low abuse potential in this group, unless there is a history of substance abuse; therefore, assessment for aberrant drug-related behavior among chronic pain patients is important to manage these patients with opioid therapy properly.

The prevalence of drug abuse, dependence, or addiction in chronic pain patients ranges from approximately 3 to 19% [44]. Yet, addictive disorders occur in approximately 3–26% of the general population [45, 46] and in 40–60% of patients who suffered major trauma [47–49]. Therefore, pain physicians are likely to encounter patients with a concurrent addictive disorder. Recognizing aberrant drug-related behavior can assist in effectively screening patients for addiction in pain treatment settings.

To refine the concept of addiction in the context of chronic pain, the American Society of Addiction Medicine, the American Pain Society, and the American Academy of Pain Medicine agreed on the following definition that supports our neurobiologic and psychologic understanding of addiction [50]: '[Addiction is] a primary, chronic, neurobiologic disease with genetic, psychosocial, and environmental factors influencing its development and manifestations. It is characterized by behaviors that include one or more of the following: impaired control over drug use, continued use despite harm, compulsive use, and craving'. In order to treat pain effectively, aberrant drug-related behavior should be noted, and addiction should be addressed concurrently.

In assessing for addiction during opioid use, the clinician should collect the patient's personal and family history of substance abuse as well as relevant objective information from the physical examination, observation, and laboratory tests. The clinician should also use appropriate screening instruments, such as the CAGE-AID [51].

When treating patients with opioids for long periods of time, it is important to follow them regularly and identify behavior suggestive of addiction. Behavior that should prompt investigation includes: continued use of drugs despite adverse consequences or harm secondary to use, loss of control over drug use, and preoccupation with use due to craving. A pattern of such behavior, rather than intermittent manifestation of one or two of these actions, warrants further assessment. Further examination into each behavior will assist in identifying key features of aberrant behavior.

The beneficial effects of opioids may be hindered by the phenomenon of tolerance. Patients deriving benefit from opioids should experience a reduction in pain and maintenance or improvement of function in areas such as relationships, work, sleep, and mood. When using opioids improperly, however, patients tend to develop impaired psychosocial functioning. For instance, addicted patients tend to lose function in critical aspects of life relating to their jobs, friendships, mood, and familial relationships. Consequently, patients being treated with opioids who persist in their disability or experience deterioration in the functional activities of living despite rehabilitative support may suffer from addiction or substance abuse. Likewise, changes in mental status or intoxication from opioids may reflect a desire for the euphoric reward of the medication rather than a need for its analgesic benefit. Tolerance to the analgesic effects of opioids does not develop quickly in patients receiving the medication properly for pain [52]. Tolerance to opioid-induced euphoria, however, does develop rapidly, necessitating higher doses to achieve the same effect. Patients with active addiction thus tend to escalate the dose of opioid to attain this euphoric state [53]. This pattern of behavior probably highlights an addictive response to the opioid in a way that promotes continued use of the drug despite adverse consequences.

Of course, pain specialists should consider other possible causes of aberrant behavior such as pseudoaddiction, i.e., drug-seeking behavior due to inadequate dosage of opioid [54], opioid-resistant pain, continual sedation at analgesic doses, and opioid-induced hyperalgesia. Recognizing patterns of aberrant behaviors, rather than isolated behaviors, will aid in assessing for addiction.

Compulsive use of opioids leads to a loss of control over drug use and represents addictive behavior. In this circumstance, patients lose control over medication use due to an intense craving for the substance. In the context of treating chronic pain, patients may overuse opioids and request early prescription refills. Such patients may report theft or loss of medications, pills falling into the toilet or down the drain, or pets consuming opioid prescriptions. Indeed, these excuses may indicate impaired control over opioid medications. Patients may also impute overuse of opioids to inadequate treatment of pain and display withdrawal symptoms at the appointment because they have depleted the opioid supply in advance. While these circumstances may occasionally occur in patients using opioids properly, a pattern of such aberrant behavior should raise concern about addiction.

When assessing for possible addiction in chronic pain patients receiving opioids, it is important to examine a preoccupation with drug use due to craving. Many patients who receive opioids for chronic pain understandably desire continual relief of pain through an uninterrupted supply of opioids. Such patients may show intense interest in maintaining regular availability of opioids to ensure analgesia and forestall withdrawal. Further, they may inquire about the physician's vacation plans or demand reminders about clinic hours. Though this behavior does not indicate addiction, it may suggest an addictive response to opioids if the patient fails to comply with other treatment modalities. For instance, the pain specialist should confirm whether the patient actively participates in physical therapy, occupational therapy, and cognitive behavioral interventions, takes adjuvant medications, and appears amenable to considering other strategies for managing pain. If patients display no interest in applying nonopioid approaches to their analgesic regimen, then their preoccupation with opioid use suggests addiction.

If the pain specialist does not detect a pattern of aberrant behavior, he or she can be fairly confident that the patient does not suffer from an active addictive disorder. In general, patients in the pain treatment setting who comply with recommended interventions, report meaningful pain relief from opioid therapy, use opioids as prescribed, and improve their functional capacity are likely responding to the medications appropriately and not engaging in addictive behavior. Although patterns of positive behavior support the proper use of opioids, growing evidence reveals that monitoring behavior without confirmatory urine toxicology screening may fail to detect opioid misuse. For instance, both Katz and Fanicullo [55] and Belgrade [56] found that self-reports of inappropriate drug use among chronic pain patients correlated poorly with urine toxicology findings. In short, incorporating observed patterns of behavior, interviews with significant others, review of medical records, and urine toxicology monitoring can improve patient management with chronic opioid therapy.

## Depression

Many physicians have argued that chronic opioid therapy increases depressed mood and disability. Yet few studies demonstrate such a correlation. An examination of the relationship between chronic pain and depression may permit a more thorough understanding of the influence of depression on patients suffering from chronic pain.

Depression seems to be a pervasive component of chronic pain [57]. In fact, patients with chronic pain and depression tend to report greater pain intensity, greater disability, decreased activity levels, poor adjustment, and poor treatment outcome compared with chronic pain patients who are not depressed [58]. Yet, the literature fails to describe the extent to which chronic pain and depression coexist, whether a causal relationship exists, or the mechanism through which depression and pain intermingle.

The reported prevalence of depression among chronic pain patients ranges from 10 to 100% [59, 60]. Such variability probably stems from inconsistencies in defining a case as well as from variability in assessment methods for depression. Depression rates may include patients with major depressive disorder (MDD), depressive symptoms, or affective disorders like dysthymia or adjustment disorder. Hence, only some of the studies report accurate rates of depression based on standardized diagnostic criteria. Overlapping symptomatology between depression and chronic pain further complicates the accurate assessment of depression in this population. For instance, chronic pain symptoms, such as loss of energy, sleep disturbance, and appetite and weight changes, are also diagnostic features of MDD.

Several authors estimate that 30–54% of outpatient chronic pain patients suffer from MDD [61, 62]. This exceeds the current (5%) and lifetime (17%) prevalence estimates for MDD in the general population [63]. In comparing depression rates in chronic pain with other chronic medical conditions, Banks and Kerns [64] were unable to make a definitive conclusion that MDD is more common in patients suffering with chronic pain than in other chronic medical populations. They did conclude, however, that empirical data supported the notion that higher depression rates exist among patients with chronic pain. A growing body of empirical evidence from retrospective studies suggests that chronic pain leads to depression [65, 66].

Magni et al. [67] conducted a longitudinal study of 2,324 patients with musculoskeletal pain to determine whether pain predicts depressive symptoms or vice versa. They found that pain is the strongest predictor of depression in comparison with other demographic variables. The researchers hypothesized that certain pain states may be more likely to elicit depression, though depression may also be associated with the onset of specific types of pain.

The observation that a greater proportion of patients with chronic pain may develop MDD than of those with other chronic medical conditions suggests that a component of the pain syndrome accounts for the higher comorbidity. Banks and Kerns [64] proposed that chronic pain patients may think and behave differently in response to pain and that this modulation of thought may elicit depression. Specifically, the way in which a patient in chronic pain processes the pain experience (changes in life activities, duration, controllability, severity, or suffering) may predispose him/her to depression. Other factors that may contribute to depression in chronic pain patients include the type of behavior exhibited by the patient in pain as well as the response given by others to the patient's pain behavior.

## Cognitive Dysfunction

Concern about potential cognitive impairment is one of the main reasons for limiting the use of opioids in the elderly. The available research has not demonstrated deleterious effects on neuropsychological testing or EEG except in patients who were prescribed multiple types of medications, especially sedatives and hypnotics [68, 69]. Data on the cognitive side effects of opioid therapy indicate short-term effects on some aspects of cognitive functioning, but few long-term effects once stable dosing is achieved. However, a number of methodological issues weaken the strength of these conclusions and further study is warranted, particularly in specific populations, such as the elderly [70]. Studies examining cognitive side effects of opioids generally fall into two classes: short-term exposure under laboratory or clinical conditions and long-term, stable dosing under clinical conditions. Studies of short-term exposure indicate few deleterious effects of morphine [71–73] but suggest cognitive declines may occur following short-term exposure to hydromorphone [72]. Clinical trial data indicate slight reductions in memory, but no change in attention or concentration, following 6 weeks of treatment with sustained-release morphine in patients with chronic pain [74]. Other studies suggest that improvements in cognitive function may occur when pain is reduced with opioids, [75, 76] even low-dose opioids [14]. However, patients in these studies were generally young (mean age 40 years) and benefits were not observed in a very small group of patients greater than 60 years [76]. A recent report from our group indicates that controlled-release morphine is not associated with significant cognitive deficits in an elderly population with postherpetic neuralgia [15].

## Conclusion

Recent controlled clinical trials provide evidence that opioids are effective in treating most chronic pain states, malignant and nonmalignant, over a period of several weeks. Additional studies, however, are needed to determine if these opioid analgesic effects persist over longer periods of drug therapy. Three factors influence opioid responsiveness in the chronic pain population: patient-centered characteristics, pain-centered characteristics, and drug-centered characteristics. Applying these concepts to the use of opioids in treating chronic pain can help achieve maximum pain relief with limited side effects. Studies on the analgesic efficacy of NMDA antagonists in human pain states reveal both a reduction in pain (ketamine) and no difference in pain (DM). Animal studies, however, suggest a more convincing role for the use of NMDA antagonists in treating chronic pain. The abuse potential and concerns about addiction in the chronic pain population may be reduced by frequent and comprehensive assessments of aberrant behavior. The prevalence of illicit drug use in the chronic pain population may be higher than in the general population; therefore, clinicians should monitor patterns of aberrant drug behavior as well as urine toxicology results to ensure compliance with opioid treatment. Patients in chronic pain exhibit a high prevalence of MDD that demands concurrent treatment to avoid functional disability. Controversy continues over a causal relationship between chronic pain and depression; yet, clinical evidence suggests that chronic pain exacerbates depressive symptomatology.

## Acknowledgment

This study was supported in part by NIH Gant NS-26363 (SNR).

## References

1 Brookoff D: Chronic pain: A new disease? Hosp Pract 2000;7:1–18.
2 Gutstein HB, Akil H: Opioid analgesics; in Hardman JG, Limbird LL (eds): Goodman and Gilman's The Pharmacological Basis of Therapeutics, ed 10. New York, McGraw-Hill, 2001, pp 569–619.
3 Foley KM: Problems of overarching importance, which transcend organ systems; in Bennett JC, Plum F (eds): Cecil Textbook of Medicine. Philadelphia, Saunders, 1996, pp 100–107.
4 American Pain Society: Principles of Analgesic Use in the Treatment of Acute Pain and Cancer Pain, ed 4. Glenview, IL, Am Pain Soc, 1999.
5 Portenoy RK, Foley KM, Inturrisi CE: The nature of opioid responsiveness and its implications for neuropathic pain: New hypotheses derived from studies of opioid infusions. Pain 1990;43: 273–286.
6 Bruera E, MacMillan K, Hanson J, MacDonald RN: The Edmonton staging system for cancer pain: Preliminary report. Pain 1989;37:203–210.
7 Portenoy RK: Opioid tolerance and responsiveness: Research findings and clinical observations; in Gebhart GF, Hammond DL, Jensen TS (eds): Pain Research and Management: Proceedings of the 7th World Congress on Pain. Seattle, IASP Press, 1994, vol 2, pp 595–614.
8 Hanks GW: The pharmacological treatment of bone pain. Cancer Surv 1988;7:87–100.
9 Kupers RC, Konings H, Adriaensen H, Gybels JM: Morphine differentially affects the sensory and affective pain ratings in neurogenic and ideopathic forms of pain. Pain 1991;47/1:5–12.
10 Arner S, Meyerson BA: Lack of analgesic effect of opioids on neuropathic and idiopathic forms of pain. Pain 1988;33:11–23.
11 Mercadante S, Maddaloni S, Roccella S, Salvaggio L: Predictive factors in advanced cancer pain treated only by opioids. Pain 1992;50/2:151–155.
12 Galer BS, Coyle N, Pasternak GW, Portenoy RK: Individual variability in the response to different opioids: Report of five cases. Pain 1992;49:87–91.
13 Watson CP, Babul N: Efficacy of oxycodone in neuropathic pain: A randomized trial in postherpetic neuralgia. Neurology 1998;50:1837–1841.
14 Rowbotham MC, Lisa Twilling L, Davies PS, Reisner L, Taylor K, MohrD: Oral Opioid Therapy for Chronic Peripheral and Central Neuropathic Pain. N Engl J Med 2003;348:1223–1232.
15 Raja SN, Haythornthwaite JA, Pappagallo M, Clark MR, Travison TG, Sabeen S, Royall MR, Max MB: Opioids versus antidepressants in postherpetic neuralgia: A randomized, placebo-controlled trial. Neurology 2002;59:1015–1021.
16 Cherny NI, Thaler HT, Friedlander-Klar H, Lapin J, Foley KM, Houde R, Portenoy RK: Opioid responsiveness of cancer pain syndromes caused by neuropathic or nociceptive mechanisms: A combined analysis of controlled, single-dose studies. Neurology 1994;44:857–861.

17  McQuay HJ, Jadad AR, Carroll D, Faura C, Glynn CJ, Moore RA, Liu Y: Opioid sensitivity of chronic pain: A patient-controlled analgesia method. Anaesthesia 1992;47:757–767.

18  Jadad AR, Carroll D, Glynn CJ, Moore RA, McQuay HJ: Morphine responsiveness of chronic pain: Double-blind randomised crossover study with patient-controlled analgesia. Lancet 1992;339:1367–1371.

19  Benedetti F, Vighetti S, Amanzio M, Casadio C, Oliaro A, Bergamasco B, Maggi G: Dose-response relationship of opioids in nociceptive and neuropathic postoperative pain. Pain 1998;74:205–211.

20  Thomas Z, Bruera E: Use of methadone in a highly tolerant patient receiving parenteral hydromorphone. J Pain Symptom Manage 1995;10:315–317.

21  Sengupta JN, Su X, Gebhart GF: Kappa, but not mu or delta, opioids attenuate responses to distention of afferent fibers innervating the rat colon. Gastroenterology 1996;111:968–980.

22  Coderre TJ, Katz J, Vaccarino AL, Melzack R: Contribution of central neuroplasticity to pathological pain: Review of clinical and experimental evidence. Pain 1993;52:259–285.

23  Mercadante S, Portenoy RK: Opioid poorly-responsive cancer pain. 2. Basic mechanisms that could shift dose-response for analgesia. J Pain Symptom Manage 2001;21:255–264.

24  Ghorpade A, Advokat C: Evidence of a role for NMDA receptors in the facilitation of tail withdrawal after spinal transection. Pharmacol Biochem Behav 1994;48:175–181.

25  Persson J, Axelsson G, Hallin RG, Gustafsson LL: Beneficial effects of ketamine in a chronic pain state with allodynia, possibly due to central sensitization. Pain 1995;60:217–222.

26  Mercadante S, Arcuri E, Tirelli W, Casuccio A: Analgesic effect of intravenous ketamine in cancer patients on morphine therapy: A randomized, controlled, double-blind, crossover, double-dose study. J Pain Symptom Manage 2000;20:246–252.

27  Mercadante S, Portenoy RK: Opioid poorly-responsive cancer pain. 3. Clinical strategies to improve opioid responsiveness. J Pain Symptom Manage 2001;21:338–349.

28  Mercadante S, Casuccio A, Fulfaro F, Groff L, Boffi R, Villari P, Gebbia V, Ripamonti C: Switching from morphine to methadone to improve analgesia and tolerability in cancer patients: A prospective study. J Clin Oncol 2001;19:2898–2904.

29  Price DD, Mao J, Lu J, Caruso FS, Frenk H, Mayer DJ: Effects of the combined oral administration of NSAIDs and dextromethorphan on behavioral symptoms indicative of arthritic pain in rats. Pain 1996;68/1:119–127.

30  Bem JL, Peck R: Dextromethorphan: An overview of safety issues. Drug Saf 1992;7:190–199.

31  Gottschalk A, Schroeder F, Ufer M, Oncu A, Buerkle H, Standl T: Amantadine, a N-methyl-*D*-aspartate receptor antagonist, does not enhance postoperative analgesia in women undergoing abdominal hysterectomy. Anesth Analg 2001;93:192–196.

32  Heiskanen T, Hartel B, Dahl ML, Seppala T, Kalso E: Analgesic effects of dextromethorphan and morphine in patients with chronic pain. Pain 2002;96:261–267.

33  Santillan R, Maestre JM, Hurle MA, Florez J: Enhancement of opiate analgesia by nimodipine in cancer patients chronically treated with morphine: A preliminary report. Pain 1994;58:129–132.

34  Roca G, Aguilar JL, Gomar C, Mazo V, Costa J, Vidal F: Nimodipine fails to enhance the analgesic effect of slow release morphine in the early phases of cancer pain treatment. Pain 1996;68:239–243.

35  Puke MJ, Wiesenfeld-Hallin Z: The differential effects of morphine and the alpha 2 adrenoreceptor agonists clonidine and dexmedetomidine on the prevention and treatment of experimental neuropathic pain. Anesth Analg 1993;77:104–109.

36  Eisenach JC, DuPen S, Dubois M, Miguel R, Allin D: Epidural clonidine analgesia for intractable cancer pain. The Epidural Clonidine Study Group. Pain 1995;61:391–399.

37  Stevens C, Yaksh T: Opioid and adrenergic spinal receptor systems and pain control. NIDA Res Monogr 1988;81:343–352.

38  Xu XJ, Puke MJ, Wiesenfeld-Hallin Z: The depressive effect of intrathecal clonidine on the spinal flexor reflex is enhanced after sciatic nerve section in rats. Pain 1992;51:145–152.

39  Levine JD, Gordon NC, Taiwo YO, Coderre TJ: Potentiation of pentazocine analgesia by low-dose naloxone. J Clin Invest 1988;82:1574–1577.

40  Gan TJ, Ginsberg B, Glass PS, Fortney J, Jhaveri R, Perno R: Opioid-sparing effects of a low-dose infusion of naloxone in patient-administered morphine sulfate. Anesthesiology 1997;87:1075–1081.

Opioids in Chronic Pain

41    Joshi GP, Duffy L, Chehade J, Wesevich J, Gajraj N, Johnson ER: Effects of prophylactic nalmefene on the incidence of morphine-related side effects in patients receiving intravenous patient-controlled analgesia. Anesthesiology 1999;90:1007–1011.

42    Portenoy RK: Opioid therapy for chronic nonmalignant pain: A review of the critical issues. J Pain Symptom Manage 1996;11:203–217.

43    Portenoy RK: Chronic opioid therapy in nonmalignant pain. J Pain Symptom Manage 1990;5: S46–S62.

44    Fishbain DA, Rosomoff HL, Rosomoff RS: Drug abuse, dependence, and addiction in chronic pain patients. Clin J Pain 1992;8:77–85.

45    Regier DA, Myers JK, Kramer M, Robins LN, Blazer DG, et al: The NIMH Epidemiological Catchment Area Study. Arch Gen Psychiatry 1984;41:934–958.

46    Vailliant G: The Natural History of Alcoholism. Cambridge, Harvard University Press, 1984.

47    Heinemann AW, Keen M, Donohue R, Schnoll S: Alcohol use by persons with recent spinal cord injury. Arch Phys Med Rehabil 1988;69:619–624.

48    Honkanen R, Ertama L, Kuosmanen P, Linnoila M, Alha A, Visuri T: The role of alcohol in accidental falls. J Stud Alcohol 1983;44:231–245.

49    Reyna TM, Hollis HW Jr, Hulsebus RC: Alcohol related trauma. The surgeon's responsibility. Ann Surg 1985;201:194–199.

50    Definitions Related to the Use of Opioids for the Treatment of Pain: A consensus document from the American Academy of Pain Medicine, the American Pain Society, and the American Society of Addiction Medicine. http://www.ampainsoc.org/advocacy/opioids2.htm

51    Brown RL, Rounds LA: Conjoint screening questionnaire for alcohol and drug abuse. Wisc Med J 1995;94:135–140.

52    Melzack R: The tragedy of needless pain. Sci Am 1990;262:27–33.

53    Weaver M, Schnoll S: Abuse liability in opioid therapy for pain treatment in patients with an addiction history. Clin J Pain 2002;18:S61–S69.

54    Weissman DE, Haddox JD: Opioid pseudoaddiction: An iatrogenic syndrome. Pain 1989;36: 363–366.

55    Katz N, Fanciullo GJ: Role of urine toxicology testing in the management of chronic opioid therapy. Clin J Pain 2002;18:S76–S82.

56    Belgrade M: Urine toxicology testing in patients with chronic pain (abstract). American Pain Society Annual Meeting, Phoenix, 2001.

57    Fishbain DA, Cutler R, Rosomoff HL, Rosomoff RS: Chronic pain-associated depression: Antecedent or consequence of chronic pain? Clin J Pain 1997;13:116–137.

58    Davis PJ, Reeves JL 2nd, Hastie BA, Graff-Radford SB, Naliboff BD: Depression determines illness conviction and pain impact: A structural equation modeling analysis. Pain Med 2000;1: 238–244.

59    Pilowsky I, Chapman CR, Bonica JJ: Pain, depression, and illness behavior in a pain clinic population. Pain 1977;4:183–192.

60    Romano JM, Turner JA: Chronic pain and depression: Does the evidence support a relationship? Psychol Bull 1985;97:18–34.

61    Ahles TA, Khan SA, Yunus MB, Spiegel DA, Masi AT: Psychiatric status of patients with primary fibromyalgia, patients with rheumatoid arthritis, and subjects without pain: A blind comparison of DSM-III diagnoses. Am J Psychiatry 1991;148:1721–1726.

62    Haythornthwaite JA, Sieber WJ, Kerns RD: Depression and the chronic pain experience. Pain 1991;46:177–184.

63    Kessler RC, Nelson CB, McGonagle KA, Liu J, Swartz M, Blazer DG: Comorbidity of DSM-III-R major depressive disorder in the general population: Results from the US National Comorbidity Survey. Br J Psychiatry Suppl 1996;30:17–30.

64    Banks SM, Kerns RD: Explaining high rates of depression in chronic pain: A diathesis-stress framework. Psychol Bull 1996;119:95–110.

65    Gamsa A: Is emotional disturbance a precipitator or a consequence of chronic pain? Pain 1990;42:183–195.

66    Gaskin ME, Greene AF, Robinson ME, Geisser ME: Negative affect and the experience of chronic pain. J Psychosom Res 1992;36:707–713.

67　Magni G, Moreschi C, Rigatti-Luchini S, Merskey H: Prospective study on the relationship between depressive symptoms and chronic musculoskeletal pain. Pain 1994;56:289–297.

68　McNairy SL, Maruta T, Ivnik RJ, Swanson DW, Ilstrup DM: Prescription medication dependence and neuropsychologic function. Pain 1984;18:169–177.

69　Ziegler DK: Opiate and opioid use in patients with refractory headache. Cephalalgia 1994; 14:5–10.

70　Ebly EM, Hogan DB, Fung TS: Potential adverse outcomes of psychotropic and narcotic drug use in Canadian seniors. J Clin Epidemiol 1997;50:857–863.

71　Hanks GW, O'Neill WM, Simpson P, Wesnes K: The cognitive and psychomotor effects of opioid analgesics. II. A randomized controlled trial of single doses of morphine, lorazepan and placebo in healthy subjects. Eur J Clin Pharmacol 1995;48:455–460.

72　Rapp SE, Egan KJ, Ross BK, Wild LM, Terman GW, Ching JM: A multidimensional comparison of morphine and hydromorphone patient-controlled analgesia. Anesth Analg 1996;82:1043–1048.

73　Zacny JP, Conley K, Marks S: Comparing the subjective, psychomotor and physiological effects of intravenous nalbuphine and morphine in healthy volunteers. J Pharmacol Exp Ther 1997;280: 1159–1169.

74　Moulin DE, Iezzi A, Amireh R, Sharpe WKJ, Boyd D, Merskey H: Randomised trial of oral morphine for chronic non-cancer pain. Lancet 1996;347:143–147.

75　Tassain V, Attal N, Fletcher D, Brasseur L, Degieux P, Chauvin M, Bouhassira D: Long term effects of oral sustained release morphine on neuropsychological performance in patients with chronic non-cancer pain. Pain 2003;104:389–400.

76　Jamison RN, Schein JR, Vallow S, Ascher S, Vorsanger GJ, Katz NP: Neuropsychological effects of long-term opioid use in chronic pain patients. J Pain Symptom Manage 2003;26:913–921.

Paul J. Christo, MD
Division of Pain Medicine,
Department of Anesthesiology and Critical Care Medicine
Johns Hopkins University School of Medicine
550 N. Broadway, Suite 301, Baltimore, MD 21205 (USA)
Tel. +1 410 955 1818, Fax +1 410 502 6730, E-Mail pchristo@jhmi.edu

Clark MR, Treisman GJ (eds): Pain and Depression. An Interdisciplinary Patient-Centered Approach. Adv Psychosom Med. Basel, Karger, 2004, vol 25, pp 138–150

...........................

# Opioid Prescribing for Chronic Nonmalignant Pain in Primary Care: Challenges and Solutions

*Yngvild Olsen*[a], *Gail L. Daumit*[a–d]

[a]Division of General Internal Medicine, Department of Medicine, Johns Hopkins University School of Medicine, [b]Welch Center for Prevention, Epidemiology, and Clinical Research, Johns Hopkins University School of Medicine and Bloomberg School of Public Health and Departments of [c]Health Policy and Management and [d]Epidemiology, Johns Hopkins University, Bloomberg School of Public Health, Baltimore, Md., USA

## Abstract

Evaluating and treating patients with chronic nonmalignant pain, especially with opioid medications, often causes discomfort on the part of primary care physicians. A number of patient-, physician-, and system-related issues converge to make treating chronic pain a complex matter. Patient-related issues include an inability to define a clear anatomic cause for patients' pain, comorbid psychiatric conditions, and past and current substance abuse. Physicians lack training on the appropriate evaluation and treatment of chronic nonmalignant pain, fear creating addicts, and often face intense pharmaceutical industry pressure to prescribe medications. A paucity of practical clinical practice guidelines, controversy over the effectiveness of opioids on chronic nonmalignant pain, and concern about potential legal and regulatory ramifications add to the complexity of caring for these patients. Possible multifaceted solutions exist to minimize provider discomfort and improve their ability to treat patients appropriately. Examples include comprehensive, practical multidimensional guidelines on the evaluation and treatment of chronic nonmalignant pain, Web-based teleconferenced consultations with subspecialists, reduced pharmaceutical pressure, enhanced continuing medical education and pregraduate training, multispecialty coordinated care of patients with adequate reimbursement for such care, and physician access to state-based systems to track opioid prescriptions.

## Introduction

Office-based physicians encounter pain, whether acute or chronic, on a daily basis [1]. Most primary care physicians (PCPs) do not have difficulty managing acute pain – evaluating, locating, and treating causes of acute pain is what their medical training best prepares them to do. The epidemiology of chronic nonmalignant pain in primary care, however, dictates that physicians also need to know how to manage this common problem. The World Health Organization, in a large, cross-national survey, estimated that the prevalence of persistent pain in primary care settings ranges from 5.5 to 33% [2]. Other researchers in smaller studies of patients and physicians in primary care offices have documented prevalence rates of 11–45% [3–5]. Chronic pain is the leading cause of disability in the United States, with arthritis alone resulting in 750,000 hospitalizations and 36 million outpatient visits annually [6]. The Centers for Disease Control estimates that the total cost of arthritis, including lost productivity, exceeds USD 82 million per year [6].

Despite its frequency and tremendous economic and societal burden, research shows that chronic pain often goes undertreated. According to the Michigan Chronic Pain Study, in 1997, 20% of the adults in Michigan suffered from chronic pain conditions and 70% of the survey responders reported having persistent pain despite treatment [7]. An American Pain Society (APS)-sponsored survey of chronic, nonmalignant pain sufferers with moderate to severe pain found that 41% of the 805 respondents reported not having their pain under control despite medications and adjuvant therapies [8].

In managing chronic nonmalignant pain, most PCPs feel comfortable prescribing nonopioid therapies, such as all the classes of nonsteroidal anti-inflammatory drugs, Tylenol, and muscle relaxants, and nonpharmacologic treatments such as physical therapy. However, all PCPs have encountered patients for whom these medications and therapies are not enough and who require stronger medications in the form of opioids prescription. Multiple patient, physician, and system-related issues converge to make PCPs often uncomfortable about prescribing opioids for chronic nonmalignant pain (fig. 1).

## Patient-Related Issues

Patients with chronic nonmalignant pain often have no identifiable anatomic lesion that PCPs can point to as a clear cause of pain and that, in a doctor's mind, better justifies the use of long-term strong opioid medications [9]. Without objective evidence of pathology, there is less to counter the multiple forces that weigh in on the side of not prescribing opioids. If PCPs choose

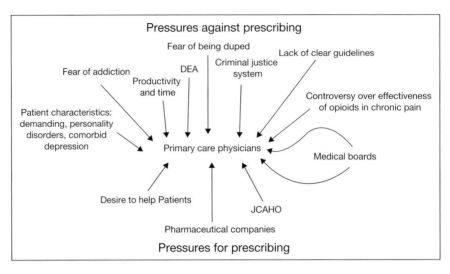

**Fig. 1.** Pressures on PCPs against and for prescribing opioids for chronic nonmalignant pain.

to prescribe opioids in these situations, they often will select short-acting opioids on an as-needed basis, a practice contrary to most pain specialists' recommended dosing schedules [10, 11].

Research has shown that chronic pain patients tend to have a higher prevalence of comorbid psychiatric disorders, such as depression [12] and borderline personality disorders [13], and that the presence of these conditions is associated with poorer pain control [14]. Within the past 20 years, PCPs have improved significantly in their treatments of depression [15], but when depression is combined with chronic pain and personality disorders, these patients often become complicated and frustrating. Prescribing opioids in these situations is something PCPs usually might try to avoid although opioids may be the appropriate treatment depending on the diagnosis, and the type and chronicity of the patient's pain. If patients feel that their pain is not adequately addressed, they may become demanding and sometimes can give the appearance of being drug-seeking or addicted when in reality they are not [16].

If patients have a history of substance abuse, then the treatment of chronic pain becomes even more difficult for PCPs. This group of patients has almost 4 times the odds of exhibiting prescription opioid abuse behaviors compared to patients without a lifetime history of substance abuse [17]. Often in these patients, however, it becomes difficult to distinguish whether the substance abuse, including prescription pain medicine addiction, came about as a consequence of chronic pain treatment or whether the substance abuse is exacerbating the chronic pain symptoms [18].

## Physician-Related Issues

Ask most physicians about why they chose their profession and you will hear the same answer – to in some way or another help people. At medical school graduations across the country, new MDs swear to some version of the Hippocratic oath, promising to live up to this responsibility. When faced with patients who demand extra time and extra attention in the midst of all the pressures PCPs face to not prescribe opioids, the Hippocratic oath may become harder to follow. Although no empiric data exists on the difference in lengths of visit in primary care settings for chronic pain patients compared to patients with other chronic diseases of similar severity, busy practitioners faced with demanding chronic pain patients may undertreat or overtreat the pain by handing patients prescriptions for various analgesics, including opioids, without taking the time to really listen to, talk with, or examine them.

The data on the addictive potential of opioid prescription drugs is variable, but the fear of creating addicts is one of the most often cited reasons why PCPs feel uncomfortable prescribing opiates [19]. The studies that have addressed this have found that 4% [20] to 31% [17] of patients without substance abuse histories seen in primary care clinics exhibit addictive behaviors with respect to their prescription pain medications. Differences in patient population and different definitions of addiction may explain the variable rates of opioid use disorders noted across these studies. Recent abuses and overdose fatalities from Oxycontin®™ have added fuel to PCPs' fears of creating addicts in managing chronic nonmalignant pain with opioids [21].

One physician-related issue not often discussed in the debate over the use of opioids by PCPs in the treatment of chronic nonmalignant pain is the fear on the part of PCPs of being duped. No one likes having the wool pulled over their eyes but PCPs pride themselves on the continuity they have with patients and the ability to develop ongoing, meaningful therapeutic relationships with their patients. If the trust developed in that relationship is broken, then PCPs may feel extremely taken advantage of, deceived, and betrayed by someone they were investing time and energy in to help. Although physicians are taught to practice according to evidence-based guidelines, experiences such as these are bound to taint PCPs' outlooks on similar patients they may encounter.

In many areas of the country, particularly rural areas, PCPs also have relatively little specialty back up to help guide them in managing difficult patients with chronic nonmalignant pain. Without such resources to turn to, PCPs are left to often conjecture when they should be using other modalities such as ultrasound or pharmacotherapies such as Neurontin, Topamax, or opioids.

Medical school and residency curricula and continuing medical education on chronic pain, its evaluation, and treatment are sorely lacking [22, 23]. Residents, faculty, and private PCPs alike bemoan the presence of 'drug-seeking' chronic pain patients on their clinic schedules, but partly this stems from their lack of knowledge about how to adequately handle these patients, how to appropriately prescribe opioids, dosing of longer-acting, stronger agents, and the latest techniques for treating chronic pain. Without confidence in their skills and ability to manage chronic nonmalignant pain, PCPs become more susceptible to the various other pressures that influence their prescribing of opioids.

## System-Related Issues

### Criminal Justice System

In February 2002, Dr. James Graves of Florida became the first physician in the country to be convicted of manslaughter for contributing to the fatal overdoses of patients by prescribing Oxycontin [24]. Prior to and following his conviction, numerous other physicians, from family physicians to pain specialists in Maine, California, Florida, and South Carolina, have been charged with racketeering, drug dealing, and manslaughter through prescribing Oxycontin to patients who subsequently died of overdoses [24–27]. PCPs understandably would feel increasingly uncomfortable even legitimately prescribing opioids if they thought they could be faced with a remote possibility of loss of their license and livelihood, jail time, or public humiliation.

However, as a civil case in California in 2001 shows, PCPs do face potential punitive consequences from their inaction. In this case, Dr. Wing Chin was found guilty of committing elder abuse and recklessness for failing to adequately treat the chronic pain of one of his patients with opioid medications [28]. These criminal and civil suits highlight potential new risks to physicians associated with managing patients with chronic pain, adding to the distress they already feel about prescribing this class of drugs.

### The Drug Enforcement Administration

In addition to fears of legal action taken against them from the criminal justice system, PCPs also face the potential of investigation and punitive actions from the Drug Enforcement Administration (DEA). In Texas, which instituted a triplicate controlled substances prescription in 1982, schedule II opioid prescriptions dropped by 64% in the year following the policy change [29]. Surveys of physicians regarding their prescribing patterns of opiate medications reveal that fear of DEA investigation is among the most frequently cited reasons for not prescribing opioids [30, 31].

## Medical Boards

Adding even further to the complicated melting pot of pressures, state medical boards create their own system of incentives and disincentives for PCPs in treating chronic nonmalignant pain with opioids. Since medical boards carry the responsibility and burden of reprimanding and sanctioning negligent physicians in each state, they carry a vested interest in the prescribing patterns of PCPs. State medical boards vary in how they carry out surveillance of physicians in this regard but in most states there is a mixed message given to PCPs – on the one hand, PCPs must treat pain adequately, using opioids if necessary, or face the consequences of potentially negligent practice but they must not overprescribe opioids or they face the consequences of potentially negligent practice [32].

## Joint Commission on Accreditation of Healthcare Organizations

In recent years, the Joint Commission on Accreditation of Healthcare Organizations (JCAHO) has on the behalf of patients actively become involved in the issue of pain treatment. Acknowledging the plight of pain sufferers and the importance of adequate pain treatment to the overall well-being of patients, the Joint Commission in 1999 announced that, as of the 2001 accreditation process, physicians were expected to assess all patients, both in inhospital as well as in ambulatory-based settings, for the presence and severity of pain and to address these complaints if present [33]. In effect, JCAHO elevated pain to the status of the fifth vital sign alongside blood pressure and heart rate [34]. Because failure to comply with these expectations could have dire consequences for the accreditation status of health care systems, PCPs working in these institutions now face added pressure from administrators to ensure that chronic pain is adequately treated without necessarily receiving guidance on how opioids fit into this.

## Pharmaceutical Companies

Pharmaceutical companies have been in the business of manufacturing therapeutic opioid medications since before the formal beginning of the industry, but not until the introduction of Oxycontin had the issue of pharmaceutical marketing of opioid drugs to physicians garnered such media attention. Pharmaceutical company representatives frequent doctor offices on a daily basis, plying their wares but many PCPs find their presence a necessary evil. Restrictions have been placed on what these representatives can and cannot do in order to entice physicians to prescribe the particular medication they are promoting [35]. However, recent lay press articles document the aggressive marketing practices of Purdue Pharma, the manufacturer of Oxycontin [36]. While many feel that these marketing tactics were excessive, they worked to convince large numbers of PCPs to prescribe Oxycontin. Beginning with its introduction in 1995, sales of Oxycontin skyrocketed and it quickly became one of the fastest selling drugs on the market [37].

### Lack of Clear Guidelines

Since the early 1990s individual pain researchers and specialty organizations have produced several disease-specific guidelines for the management of chronic nonmalignant conditions such as sickle cell anemia [19, 38–41]. In 1997 the APS issued a broad consensus statement on the use of opioids in the treatment of chronic nonmalignant pain, acknowledging the lack of clear universally accepted guidelines on this issue [42]. However, existing guidelines differ in their views on the role of opioids for patients and rather than clarifying the situation, they have added to the confusion. More recently, the APS outlined treatment guidelines for arthritis in children and adults, a first step towards clearer management guidelines for a broad category of common, chronic nonmalignant pain conditions [43].

### Controversy over the Effectiveness of Opioids in the Treatment of Chronic Nonmalignant Pain

Underlying much of the debate over the use of opioids for the treatment of chronic nonmalignant pain is the controversy over the effectiveness of these medications in improving outcomes in chronic, nonmalignant pain patients. While the trend has been towards more and more acceptability of opioids in treating chronic nonmalignant pain, few randomized controlled trials have been conducted to definitively answer this question. Those that do exist [44–52] suggest a benefit from opioids, but follow-up is often short, leaving unclear the effects of long-term treatment with these medications.

Jamison et al. [48] conducted an open, multiphase study of 36 patients with chronic back pain in which they were followed for 16 weeks after being randomized to either naproxen, fixed-dose oxycodone, or titrated-dose oxycodone and sustained-release morphine, with a subsequent 16-week phase during which they all received titrated-dose opioids. The authors found that pain and emotional distress improved significantly more in the opioid groups compared with the naproxen only, but there were no differences noted in activity level or hours of sleep reported by patients. Roth et al. [49], in a 2-week, industry-sponsored double-blind randomized trial, found superior pain relief from sustained-release oxycodone compared with placebo in a group of patients with persistent, severe osteoarthritis pain.

Recently, Rowbotham et al. [50], in an 8-week double-blind randomized trial of 81 patients with refractory neuropathic pain, found that high-dose levorphanol produced greater pain relief than lower doses of the medication, but both dosages equally improved affective distress, interference with functioning, and sleep. There was a higher incidence of side effects in the high-dose levorphanol group.

## Possible Solutions

Given the numerous pressures on PCPs from different areas in managing chronic nonmalignant pain with opioids, the solutions to try to minimize provider discomfort and improve their ability to treat such patients appropriately also need to come from multiple angles (table 1).

First, PCPs need readily available comprehensive, practical guidelines for how to effectively and appropriately evaluate patients with chronic nonmalignant pain. Such guidelines would ideally include information on the diagnostic workup and identification of the type of pain in question (i.e. whether neuropathic, inflammatory, or musculoskeletal), and the need for a multidimensional assessment of psychiatric comorbidities, disability status, life stressors, and social supports prior to initiating any treatment. In addition, guidelines would provide the indications for opioids, appropriate follow-up of patients on these medications, sample contracts and informed consent forms that are currently being used by some PCPs, and patient information pamphlets that PCPs could provide as part of their treatment protocol. Respected and well-known agencies such as the Agency for Healthcare Research and Quality (AHRQ) could serve as the source of such guidelines.

Second, with the advent of the Internet and the availability of web-based information, organizational web sites such as that of the APS could be expanded to serve as available resources that PCPs involved in managing patients with chronic nonmalignant pain could access for information, answers to questions, or as a site for locating pain specialists in their area. As part of this, a network of pain specialists willing to serve as consultants, long distance or locally, could be compiled and distributed to PCPs nationally.

Having access to objective information on the benefits and risks of opioid medications from sources other than pharmaceutical companies should help balance any excessive marketing practices experienced by PCPs. In addition, in accordance with the American Medical Society guidelines on the use of incentives by pharmaceutical companies, PCPs should report any unethical behavior that they are subject to or witness on the part of pharmaceutical company representatives.

***Table 1.*** Possible solutions to lessen PCP discomfort in prescribing opioids for chronic nonmalignant pain

Readily available comprehensive, practical guidelines on management of chronic nonmalignant pain, including diagnostic evaluation, multidimensional psychosocial assessment, and treatment approaches based on diagnostic formulations

Availability of web-based resource sites such as the APS to access information and advice, and to locate local pain specialists

Network of willing pain specialists to serve as local or long-distance consultants

Increased reliance on nonpharmaceutical sources for information on risks and benefits of opioids in the management of chronic nonmalignant pain

Increased education on the management of chronic nonmalignant pain with opioids through enhanced continuing medical education courses, conferences, and specialty pain organizations

Required continuing medical education credits in the management of chronic nonmalignant pain, including appropriate use of opioids

Inclusion of chronic pain and opioid prescribing curricula in medical school and residency training

Improved links of communication between PCPs and other health care providers involved in the care of patients with chronic nonmalignant pain on opioids

Access to state-maintained opioid-prescribing database information for verification of patient adherence to opioid treatment

In addition to enhancing available resources for PCPs, strengthening their own knowledge around the management of chronic nonmalignant pain, including the appropriate prescribing of opioids, would likely alleviate much of their discomfort in this area. For practicing providers, continuing medical education programs and courses offered either through individual state medical boards, specialized organizations such as the APS, or through conferences held by large medical centers would provide acceptable venues in which PCPs could learn the practical skills of how to manage chronic nonmalignant pain. In order to ensure that providers maintain a minimum set of skills with regard to chronic pain management and the use of opioids, the American Board of Internal Medicine and state licensing boards should require that PCPs obtain a certain number of continuing medical education credits per year in this area, as is done in California [53]. Continuing medical education courses should provide comprehensive, practical information on the diagnostic evaluation of chronic nonmalignant pain, the identification of the type of pain, obtaining a multidimensional psychosocial history from patients prior to planning treatment, and review the available and appropriate treatment approaches based on a diagnostic formulation.

Physician education on this topic, however, should begin before providers are fully trained. The American College of Graduate Medical Education should call for the inclusion of chronic pain curricula in medical schools and residency programs and residents should be expected to demonstrate competency in this area. Central to these curricula would be the importance of diagnosis and a comprehensive multidimensional psychosocial evaluation prior to treatment, and appropriate prescribing of opioid medications and follow-up of patients on such therapies.

While not always deliberate, patients with chronic nonmalignant pain conditions on prescription opioids often end up with a multispecialty team of health care providers involved in their care – PCPs, pharmacists, physical therapists, pain specialists, and often psychiatrists. In order to maximize the effectiveness of each individual provider's care and minimize the negative aspects of opioid treatment, providers need to improve communication between them and ideally coordinate care as if they were a deliberately put together multispecialty team. Not only will this streamline and potentially improve care for patients, it will also offer a source of support and a resource for the providers caring for an often challenging population. It will also ensure that patients receive the appropriate treatment given their specific diagnosis, type of pain, and any psychiatric comorbidities or life stressors that may make treatment more challenging. Third-party payers should recognize the importance of multispecialty care by adequately reimbursing PCPs and others for providing these types of services.

In lieu of an actual team-based approach to caring for patients with chronic nonmalignant pain on prescription opioids, several states, including Utah, maintain confidential records that track opioid prescriptions across the state [54]. Primary care providers that prescribe opioids for chronic nonmalignant pain may obtain, with informed consent from the patient, information from the state database on the number of opioid prescriptions a certain patient has had filled within a certain period of time, which other providers have provided similar prescriptions, and how many emergency department visits the patient has had. This information is then used to verify adherence to the treatment procedure that is defined by the PCP and agreed upon by the patient prior to initiating opioid medications.

## Conclusion

In 1998 the Federation of State Medical Boards issued model guidelines for the use of opioids in the treatment of pain, stating 'all physicians should become knowledgeable about effective methods of pain treatment as well as statutory requirements for prescribing controlled substances' [32]. A multitude of contradictory forces currently exert pressure on PCPs in their decision to treat or not to treat chronic nonmalignant pain with opioid medications. These points of pressure combine to create a great deal of discomfort and unease on the part of PCPs in managing these patients and prescribing opioids, which ultimately may impact the care that these patients receive. However, solutions exist to minimize the unease felt by PCPs and provide them with the confidence necessary to manage chronic nonmalignant pain and the appropriate use of opioid medications. Given the epidemiology of chronic pain, the aging of the population, and the role of the PCP, it is imperative that we stand up to the challenge.

## References

1   Fox C, Berger D, Fine PG, Gebhart GF, Grabois M, Kulich RJ, Lande SD, McCarberg B, Portenoy R: Pain Assessment and Treatment in the Managed Care Environment. http:// www.ampainsoc.org/managedcare/pdf/aps_position.pdf. 3-11-2003.
2   Gureje O, Von Korff M, Simon GE, Gater R: Persistent pain and well-being: A World Health Organization Study in Primary Care. JAMA 1998;280/2:147–151.
3   Kumpusalo E, Mantyselka P, Takala J: Chronic pain in primary care. Fam Pract 2000;17:352.
4   Croft P, Rigby AS, Boswell R, Schollum J, Silman A: The prevalence of chronic widespread pain in the general population. J Rheumatol 1993;20:710–713.
5   Elliott AM, Smith BH, Penny KI, Smith WC, Chambers WA: The epidemiology of chronic pain in the community. Lancet 1999;354:1248–1252.
6   Centers for Disease Control and Prevention: Targeting Arthritis: The Nation's Leading Cause of Disability 2003. http://www.cdc.gov/nccdphp/aag/pdf/aag_arthritis2003.pdf.
7   EPIC/MRA: Michigan Chronic Pain Survey. American Pain Society Bulletin, 2000.
8   Roper Starch Worldwide, Inc: Chronic Pain in America: Roadblocks to Relief. http:// www.ampainsoc.org/whatsnew/toc_road.htm#toc.
9   Gallagher RM: Primary care and pain medicine. A community solution to the public health problem of chronic pain. Med Clin North Am 1999;83:555–583.
10  Grossman S, Sheidler V: Cancer pain; in Abeloff MD (ed): Clinical Oncology. New York, Churchill Livingstone, 2000, pp 544–547.
11  McCarberg BH, Barkin RL: Long-acting opioids for chronic pain: Pharmacotherapeutic opportunities to enhance compliance, quality of life, and analgesia. Am J Ther 2001;8/3:181–186.
12  Fishbain DA, Cutler R, Rosomoff HL, Rosomoff RS: Chronic pain-associated depression: Antecedent or consequence of chronic pain? A review. Clin J Pain 1997;13/2:116–137.
13  Sansone RA, Whitecar P, Meier BP, Murry A: The prevalence of borderline personality among primary care patients with chronic pain. Gen Hosp Psychiatry 2001;23/4:193–197.
14  Ericsson M, Poston WS, Linder J, Taylor JE, Haddock CK, Foreyt JP: Depression predicts disability in long-term chronic pain patients. Disabil Rehabil 2002;24:334–340.
15  Wittchen HU, Kessler RC, Beesdo K, Krause P, Hofler M, Hoyer J: Generalized anxiety and depression in primary care: Prevalence, recognition, and management. J Clin Psychiatry 2002; 63(suppl 8):24–34.
16  Weissman DE, Haddox JD: Opioid pseudoaddiction – An iatrogenic syndrome. Pain 1989;36: 363–366.
17  Reid MC, Engles-Horton LL, Weber MB, Kerns RD, Rogers EL, O'Connor PG: Use of opioid medications for chronic noncancer pain syndromes in primary care. J Gen Intern Med 2002;17: 173–179.

18    Fishbain DA, Rosomoff HL, Rosomoff RS: Drug abuse, dependence, and addiction in chronic pain patients. Clin J Pain 1992;8/2:77–85.

19    Portenoy RK: Chronic opioid therapy in nonmalignant pain. J Pain Symptom Manage 1990; 5(1 suppl):S46–S62.

20    Adams NJ, Plane MB, Fleming MF, Mundt MP, Saunders LA, Stauffacher EA: Opioids and the treatment of chronic pain in a primary care sample. J Pain Symptom Manage 2001;22:791–796.

21    Albert T: Death Fuels Brouhaha over Oxycontin Prescribing Practices. www.ama-assn.org/sci-pubs/amnews/pick_01/prsc0820.htm. 3-16-2003.

22    Margolis RB, Zimny GH, Miller D, Taylor JM: Internists and the chronic pain patient. Pain 1984;20/2:151–156.

23    Turk DC, Brody MC, Okifuji EA: Physicians' attitudes and practices regarding the long-term prescribing of opioids for non-cancer pain. Pain 1994;59/2:201–208.

24    Kaczor B: US FL: Panhandle Doctor's OxyContin Conviction to Send Message. http://www.mapinc.org/drugnews/v02/n298/a11.html. 3-16-2003.

25    Meier B: Oxycontin prescribers face charges in fatal overdoses. New York Times, Jan 19, 2002, sect A, column 1:14.

26    Albert T, Adams D: OxyContin Crackdown Raises Physician, Patient Concerns. http://www.ama-assn.org/sci-pubs/amnews/pick_01/prl10625.htm. 3-16-2003.

27    Mishra R: US ME: Painkiller tears through Maine. Boston Globe, Mar 23, 2001.

28    Okie S: California jury finds doctor negligent in managing pain. Washington Post, June 15, 2001, sect A: A02.

29    Angarola RT, Joranson DE: State controlled-substance laws and pain control. APS Bull 1992;2/3: 10–15.

30    Hill CS Jr: Relationship among cultural, educational, and regulatory agency influences on optimum cancer pain treatment. J Pain Symptom Manage 1990;5(1 suppl):S37–S45.

31    Clark HW, Sees KL: Opioids, chronic pain, and the law. J Pain Symptom Manage 1993;8/5:297–305.

32    The Federation of State Medical Boards of the United States Inc: Model Guidelines for the Use of Controlled Substances for the Treatment of Pain. http://www.fsmb.org/. 4-2-2003.

33    Dahl J: New JCAHO standards focus on pain management. Oncol Issues 1999;14:27–28.

34    American Pain Society: Pain: The Fifth Vital Sign. http://www.ampainsoc.org/advocacy/fifth.htm. 4-2-2003.

35    Gifts to Physicians Work Group: Gifts to Physicians from Industry. http://www.ama-assn.org/ama/pub/article/4001-4236.html. 4-2-2003.

36    Meier B, Petersen M: Sales of painkiller grew rapidly, but success brought a high cost. New York Times, Mar 5, 2001, sect A, column 1:1.

37    Adams C: Painkiller's sales far exceeded levels anticipated by maker. Wall Street Journal, May 16, 2002.

38    Practice guidelines for chronic pain management. A report by the American Society of Anesthesiologists Task Force on Pain Management, Chronic Pain Section. Anesthesiology 1997; 86:995–1004.

39    Schofferman J: Long-term use of opioid analgesics for the treatment of chronic pain of nonmalignant origin. J Pain Symptom Manage 1993;8/5:279–288.

40    Benjamin LJ, Dampier CC, Jacox AK, et al: Guideline for the Management of Acute and Chronic Pain in Sickle-Cell Disease. IAPS Clinical Practice Guideline Series No 11. Glenview, American Pain Society, 1999.

41    Hagen N, Flynne P, Hays H, MacDonald N: Guidelines for managing chronic non-malignant pain. Opioids and other agents. College of Physicians and Surgeons of Alberta. Can Fam Physician 1995;41:49–53.

42    The use of opioids for the treatment of chronic pain. A consensus statement from the American Academy of Pain Medicine and the American Pain Society. Clin J Pain 1997;13/1:6–8.

43    Arthritis Pain Guideline Panel: Guideline for the Management of Pain in Osteoarthritis, Rheumatoid Arthritis, and Juvenile Chronic Arthritis, ed 2. Glenview, American Pain Society, 2002.

44    Arkinstall W, Sandler A, Goughnour B, Babul N, Harsanyi Z, Darke AC: Efficacy of controlled-release codeine in chronic non-malignant pain: A randomized, placebo-controlled clinical trial. Pain 1995;62/2:169–178.

45 Allan L, Hays H, Jensen NH, de Waroux BL, Bolt M, Donald R, et al: Randomised crossover trial of transdermal fentanyl and sustained release oral morphine for treating chronic non-cancer pain. BMJ 2001;322:1154–1158.

46 Dellemijn PL, Vanneste JA: Randomised double-blind active-placebo-controlled crossover trial of intravenous fentanyl in neuropathic pain. Lancet 1997;349:753–758.

47 Moulin DE, Iezzi A, Amireh R, Sharpe WK, Boyd D, Merskey H: Randomised trial of oral morphine for chronic non-cancer pain. Lancet 1996;347:143–147.

48 Jamison RN, Raymond SA, Slawsby EA, Nedeljkovic SS, Katz NP: Opioid therapy for chronic noncancer back pain. A randomized prospective study. Spine 1998;23:2591–2600.

49 Roth SH, Fleischmann RM, Burch FX, Dietz F, Bockow B, Rapoport RJ, et al: Around-the-clock, controlled-release oxycodone therapy for osteoarthritis-related pain: Placebo-controlled trial and long-term evaluation. Arch Intern Med 2000;160:853–860.

50 Rowbotham MC, Twilling L, Davies PS, Reisner L, Taylor K, Mohr D: Oral opioid therapy for chronic peripheral and central neuropathic pain. N Engl J Med 2003;348:1223–1232.

51 Watson CP, Babul N: Efficacy of oxycodone in neuropathic pain: A randomized trial in postherpetic neuralgia. Neurology 1998;50:1837–1841.

52 Wilder-Smith CH, Hill L, Spargo K, Kalla A: Treatment of severe pain from osteoarthritis with slow-release tramadol or dihydrocodeine in combination with NSAID's: A randomised study comparing analgesia, antinociception and gastrointestinal effects. Pain 2001;91/1–2:23–31.

53 Aroner: Section 2241.7. AB 487. Business and Professions Code. 3-27-2001.

54 United States General Accounting Office: Prescription Drugs: State Monitoring Programs Provide Useful Tool to Reduce Diversion, Washington, 2002.

Yngvild Olsen
Johns Hopkins University School of Medicine
1830 Building, Room 8012
1830 East Monument St, Baltimore, MD 21287 (USA)
Tel. +1 410 614 6440, Fax +1 410 502 6952, E-Mail yolsen@jhsph.edu

Clark MR, Treisman GJ (eds): Pain and Depression. An Interdisciplinary Patient-Centered Approach. Adv Psychosom Med. Basel, Karger, 2004, vol 25, pp 151–171

..........................

# To Help and Not to Harm: Ethical Issues in the Treatment of Chronic Pain in Patients with Substance Use Disorders

*Cynthia M.A. Geppert*

Department of Psychiatry, University of New Mexico School of Medicine and Institute for Ethics, New Mexico Health Sciences Center, Albuquerque, N.Mex., USA

## Abstract

Patients with both chronic pain and substance use disorders are increasingly encountered in a variety of treatment settings. The treatment of these patients raises a number of ethical and patient care issues. Consultation-liaison psychiatrists possess the knowledge and skills to constructively address these issues. This chapter provides clinicians with a review of clinical and ethical dilemmas related to opioid treatment of chronic pain in patients with substance use disorders. The core conflict of beneficence and nonmaleficence will be explored in relation to the concepts of autonomy, justice, respect for persons, confidentiality, and informed consent. The thesis of this discussion focuses on the clinician's desire to provide compassionate care and relieve suffering, which sometimes conflicts with the clinician's desire to improve functioning, extend longevity, and enrich quality of life. A harm reduction model for clinical decision making is summarized.

'The world is full of suffering but it is also full of the overcoming of it' – Helen Keller

## Introduction

The treatment of chronic pain in patients with substance use disorders (SUD) raises ethical issues involving principles of patient care. Even in patients without SUD there is controversy about the appropriate use of opioids for non-malignant chronic pain [1]. There is also controversy about the use of opioid agonists in treatment of addiction in persons without chronic pain [2]. These ethical questions are complicated by political and legal mandates that impact clinical judgment [3]. Further, the addiction and chronic pain communities have historically been separated in their educational, patient care, and research endeavors, with few physicians possessing the knowledge and skills in both pain and addiction medicine required to treat patients with both disorders. In an effort to address these deficits, the first joint conference on pain management and chemical dependency was held in 1996 [4].

Consultation-liaison psychiatrists are well suited to fill this gap because of their training and experience in treating both pain and addiction in a variety of settings [5]. They possess the knowledge and background to identify and constructively address the ethical dilemmas involved in caring for patients with substance use and chronic pain [6]. This chapter provides clinicians with a review of clinical and ethical issues related to opioid treatment of chronic pain in patients with SUD. The core conflict of beneficence and nonmaleficence will be explored in relation to the concepts of justice, respect for persons, informed consent, confidentiality and truth-telling. The thesis of this discussion focuses on the clinician's desire to provide compassionate care and relieve suffering, which sometimes conflicts with the clinician's desire to improve functioning, extend longevity, and enrich quality of life. A harm reduction model for clinical decision making is summarized.

## Background

The 2001 National Household Survey on Drug Abuse found that 16.6 million Americans over the age of 12 met criteria for abuse and dependence upon alcohol or illicit drugs. This figure represents an increase of 2.1 million persons when compared to 2000 estimates. The population of persons using pain medications for nonmedical purposes has steadily increased since the 1980s and now comprises an estimated 2 million people [7]. The human burden of substance use is incalculable, but the economic cost of substance abuse has been estimated at 428.1 billion in 1995. This figure includes expenditures for lost earnings from premature death and reduced job productivity as well as criminal justice and social welfare costs [8].

The epidemiology of patients suffering from chronic pain who also have SUD has not received appropriate study and the research that has been conducted has methodological problems which limit generalizability [9]. Fishbain et al. [10] reviewed 24 articles on chronic pain and alcohol and drug addiction in 1992 to ascertain the percentage of patients who met criteria for drug misuse. They identified only 7 studies with adequate methods and terminology and determined the prevalence of drug addiction/abuse/dependence was between 3.2 and 18.9%.

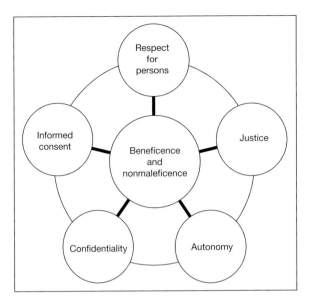

***Fig. 1.*** Hub of principles.

Conversely, the number of patients with addiction who also have chronic pain had not been adequately researched. In a recent JAMA study, Rosenblum et al. [11] looked at the prevalence and characteristics of chronic pain in 531 subjects at 13 different short-term residential SUD inpatient programs and 390 patients from two methadone maintenance programs (MMTP). Thirty-seven percent of MMTP patients and 24% of inpatients reported chronic severe pain. Further, 68% of MMTP patients and 48% of inpatients experienced levels of pain that interfered with functioning. Interestingly, among those with severe pain, inpatients (51%) were more likely than MMTP patients (34%) to have used illicit drugs to self-medicate their pain, but were less likely to be prescribed pain medications.

### Ethical Treatment of Patients with Chronic Pain

The last three decades have seen changes in the treatment of chronic pain. The recognition that clinicians underdiagnosed and undertreated pain in patients with malignancy and other terminal conditions had led to an emphasis on evaluation and treatment of pain by palliative care specialists and regulatory agencies. Treatment of malignant pain with opioids is now not only ethically acceptable but morally, and increasingly, legally, imperative (fig. 1) [12]. The medical community is increasingly viewing the treatment of nonmalignant chronic pain as ethically acceptable and there is growing regulatory acknowledgment that this is a legitimate medical practice [2, 13].

The ethical and legal position of treating chronic nonmalignant pain continues to be an area of controversy. The treatment of chronic pain in patients with current SUD or a history of addiction is a much more controversial subject upon which there is much less agreement [14]. Although there are many effective pharmacological, physical, and psychological treatments for chronic pain, a subset of patients with SUD may require opioids for adequate pain relief and acceptable quality of life. There is little scientifically conducted research regarding the risks and benefits of treating chronic pain in patients with substance abuse disorders to guide the practitioner [15, 16].

A small, mostly conceptual body of work on the ethics of treating chronic pain in patients with a current diagnosis and history of a SUD has been published. A literature search of the databases (Bioethics Line, PsychInfo and Medline) identified 5 articles dealing with the clinical or ethical issues of treating chronic pain in patients with a history of addiction or current SUD and fewer than 10 articles dealing with the ethics of nonmalignant chronic pain treatment [17–20]. One author has called this neglect of the problem of pain in the bioethics literature 'a legacy of silence' [21].


## A Common Language

The lack of clear definition of many of the terms involved in this controversy contributes to the disagreements. The terms 'addiction, dependence, tolerance, and abuse' have been widely misunderstood and misapplied even among health professionals [22]. The American Academy of Pain Medicine, American Pain Society and American Society of Addiction Medicine produced a consensus document containing definitions related to the use of opioids for treating pain [23]. The interpretation of these key terms carries ethical significance [24]. Ethical principles can help frame the clinical import of the key terms employed in scholarly and lay discussions of addiction (table 1). A shared terminology enables all professionals to educate the public about the real nature of addiction and chronic pain diagnoses and their associated pharmacological treatments.


## The Core Ethical Conflict in Chronic Pain Treatment

More than 2000 years ago, Hippocrates succinctly stated the core ethical conflict involved in the treatment of chronic pain in persons with SUD. 'I will

**Table 1.** Ethical acceptability of treating chronic pain

| Accepted | Growing consensus | Controversial |
|----------|-------------------|---------------|
| Malignant pain | Chronic nonmalignant pain | Chronic nonmalignant pain in addiction |

use my power to help the sick to the best of my ability and judgment; I will abstain from harming or wronging any man by it' [25]. Ethicists call these two obligations beneficence and nonmaleficence, literally the obligation to do good and not to do harm. Modern codes of ethics continue to regard these ancient principles as two of the physician's most basic professional obligations. The treatment of chronic pain in any patient accomplishes several recognized goals of medicine: it promotes health and prevents disease; it relieves symptoms of pain and suffering, and it improves functional status or restores previous ability to function [26].

Studies support the contention that treatment of chronic pain with opioids and other psychoactive medications in patients without a history of addiction accomplishes these goals and also may enable patients to return to work and normalize family life [27, 28]. Risk-taking behavior linked to substance abuse as well as the medical complications of addiction may lead to the development of chronic pain conditions necessitating opioid medications for adequate treatment. Between 3 and 16% of chronic pain patients have problems with drug or alcohol abuse [10, 29]. Alcohol is involved in 20% of all crashes resulting in injury. Of 936 patients admitted to a trauma unit in 1988 who had a toxicology screen, 65% were positive for more than one substance [30]. Alcohol-dependent patients are 10 times more likely to become burn victims [31].

Few studies have examined whether the benefits of long-term chronic pain therapy with opioids for chronic pain demonstrated in patients without addiction extend to patients with histories of or active SUD. A 1990 pilot study of methadone maintenance for patients with both chronic pain and substance abuse showed that 3 out of 4 patients remained in treatment for 19–21 months, stopped needle use, and/or markedly decreased substance abuse, and improved functioning despite having a psychopathology serious enough to require psychotropic medication [32]. A 2003 study of 44 patients in an integrated 10-week pain management SUD treatment found no difference between patients who continued to take opioids and those who did not during a 12-month follow-up (two thirds of the patients were opioid dependent). Both groups showed reductions in overall medication use while also reporting decreased pain. Those who continued on opioids were thought to have better functioning, suggesting a potential benefit for chronic pain medication even in patients with SUD [33].

Pain relief may actually reduce the use of alcohol and illicit drugs for self-medication, reduce craving and, thus, avoid relapse, while also increasing the probability that patients will enter or continue in addiction therapy [9]. Dunbar and Katz [34] performed a retrospective study of factors leading to prescription abuse among SUD patients treated for chronic pain for more than 1 year. Patients who were active members of groups like Alcoholics Anonymous (AA), who had a social support system, abused alcohol or had a remote history of SUD were not likely to abuse opioid therapy. Patients with poly-SUD or a prior history of abusing prescription medications were more likely to misuse medications. These studies suggest that a SUD may not be an absolute contraindication for opioid treatment for chronic nonmalignant pain. Instead, a continuum of risk must be evaluated for ethical and clinical decision making.

Historically, physicians have been apprehensive about prescribing controlled substances for patients with a history of addiction or a current SUD because of the medical, legal, and social harms that might result [35]. A study using the critical incident technique identified two common dilemmas regarding opioid use in patients with SUD. First, physicians were concerned they would cause abuse and addiction without a proper indication for opioid medication. Second, clinicians were concerned about the appropriateness of opioids for particular subtypes of pain [36]. The empirical basis and ethical cogency of these concerns must be carefully explored to ascertain their validity and importance when weighed against the substantial benefits to the patient and society from treating chronic pain. The purported risks identified in the literature are summarized in table 2.

The major risks which concern physicians prescribing opioids for patients with preexisting SUD include physical dependence, relapse to addictive behaviors, medical-legal problems for both the patient and the physician, and diminished functioning (table 3). Many clinicians equate physical dependence with addiction. Clearer understanding of the phenomena of physical dependence and tolerance may decrease suffering, unjust legal sanctions, and the costs of health care utilization and lost productivity. Many medications such as antihypertensives cause physical dependence, tolerance, and associated withdrawal symptoms [37]. Recently the pharmaceutical manufacture of paroxetine was sued because of alleged claims that the medication was 'habit-forming'; although the original ruling in favor of the plaintiff was eventually reversed, most psychopharmacologists now agree paroxetine and other short half-life antidepressants do cause a 'discontinuation' syndrome [38, 39]. Though withdrawal can adversely effect patients if improperly identified and managed, such events can easily be

**Table 2.** Ethical import of consensus definitions

| Definition | Examples of ethical significance |
|---|---|
| Addiction is a primary, chronic, neurobiologic disease, with genetic, psychosocial, and environmental factors influencing its development and manifestations; it is characterized by behaviors that include one or more of the following: impaired control over drug use, compulsive use, continued use despite harm and craving | Beneficence: recognition of true addiction can lead clinicians to obtain proper treatment of both pain and substance use<br>Informed consent: the decisional capacity and voluntarism of patients with addiction may be limited and require special consideration |
| Physical dependence is a state of adaptation that is manifested by a drug class-specific withdrawal syndrome that can be produced by abrupt cessation, rapid dose reduction, decreasing blood level of the drug, and/or administration of an antagonist | Nonmaleficence: confusion of physical dependence with addiction may lead to inadequate treatment of pain, refusal to initiate medication, or inappropriate reduction or cessation of medication<br>Justice: use of physical dependence as criteria for substance abuse and dependence unfairly singles out those using psychoactive medications |
| Tolerance is a state of adaptation in which exposure to drug induces changes that result in diminution of one or more of the drug's effects over time | Respect for persons: misunderstanding of tolerance may lead clinicians to stigmatize patients who exhibit tolerance and request additional medication<br>Confidentiality: physicians who use tolerance as a criterion for addiction may document drug addiction leading to negative psychosocial consequences for the patient |

anticipated and handled through tapering, the use of adjunctive medications, nonpharmacological therapies and judicious dose adjustments.

A second concern is that patients with a history of addiction may relapse. A person with risk factors for developing a SUD, such as certain psychiatric diagnoses or a family history of addiction, may misuse, abuse, or become dependent upon the prescribed drug [40, 41]. The rate of SUD in pain patients was from 3.2 to 18.9% in a literature review which is similar to the prevalence in the general population and represents a minority of those prescribed potentially addictive medications for pain [10]. Several assessment tools have been presented in the chronic pain literature that may assist in identifying patients who are at risk of addiction. Toxicology screening and a thorough clinical

**Table 3.** Risks of treating chronic pain in SUD

---

Biological risks
  Dependence
  Tolerance
  Withdrawal
Clinical risks: patient oriented
  New SUD
  Relapse of prior SUD
Legal risks: physician oriented
  Professional censure
  Legal sanction
Psychosocial risks: physician–patient relationship
  Manipulation of relationship
  Exploitation of the system
  Diversion of controlled substances
  Countertransference reactions

---

interview may also improve the clinician's ability to prospectively identify patients who may have or develop an addiction [42]. If these methods are used to bar patients from opioid and other effective therapies, then they may themselves cause harm to the patient [20]. If on the other hand, they are used as their authors intend, to anticipate the needs of patients with predisposition to addiction and to enable clinicians and patients to marshal other resources to support the patient during treatment, then they reduce the harms both of not treating chronic pain and of iatrogenic relapse or addiction [43].

A third issue confronting clinicians are medical-legal barriers to opioid treatment which arise in the setting of addictive drug use. Physicians fear that if they prescribe controlled substances to patients with known histories of addiction or current SUD, they may be liable to professional censure or legal sanction. Research shows this results in inadequate treatment of chronic pain in patients with SUD. Breitbart et al. [44] looked at 366 ambulatory AIDS patients in a cross-sectional study. They found that 226 of these patients reported persistent or frequent pain during the 2 weeks prior to the survey. Nearly 85% of patients with pain were receiving inadequate medication according to the Pain Management Index. Those most likely to be receiving inadequate treatment were women, less educated patients, and patients who had contracted HIV through IVDU. While physicians have some justification for their anxiety about the use of chronic opioids, there also have been legal repercussions for undertreatment of pain. A California jury found a physician guilty of elder abuse for undertreating pain [45]. The duty of a physician to treat despite legal issues has received recognition in the various physician organizations. According to the

Principles of the American Medical Association, 'A physician shall respect the law and also recognize a responsibility to seek changes in those requirements that are contrary to the best interests of the patient' [46]. Implicit in this charge is that a physician's clinical judgment be informed by an accurate, up-to-date knowledge of federal and state legislation relevant to the prescription of controlled substances in patients with addiction. This enjoins physicians to be invested in political action that will influence policy that undermines good medical practice.

The use of chronic opioids has a profound influence on behavior. The reinforcing effects of opioids may have the effect of exacerbating disability and worsening relationships for patients. The ethical intent of opioid prescribing must be to improve prosocial functioning, including behavior related to the clinical encounter. This becomes most clear when the patient develops behaviors that disrupt the doctor–patient relationship. The critical incident study referred to earlier found that physicians experienced the ethical dilemmas surrounding opioid prescription as stressful encounters that had a negative impact on self-esteem and represented a failure in the physician-patient relationship [36]. Patients who display problematic behavior, such as lying to physicians about illicit drug use or doctor shopping, trigger countertransference reactions of frustration, resentment, and fear of being manipulated [47]. These reactions are well documented in the difficult patient literature and are a long-established field of expertise for consultation-liaison psychiatry [48]. Pain specialists and primary care physicians who provide the majority of chronic pain treatment often do not have the training to manage these behaviors [49]. Physicians who experience ethical dilemmas regarding prescription of controlled substances have identified education in the pharmacology of pain management, addiction treatment, and communication skills as crucial to constructively managing countertransference reactions and maintaining the integrity of the physician–patient relationship [36].

The much quoted discussion of pseudoaddiction of Weissman and Haddox [50] underscores this point. Patients with or without a history of addiction, who receive inadequate pain medication, may respond with 'pseudoaddictive behaviors' such as unauthorized dosage increases and/or visiting multiple physicians leading physicians to suspect abuse and perhaps reduce medication, creating a vicious cycle. Responding to addictive behaviors in pain patients as if they were addicts can deprive the patient of the benefits of effective pain medication and cause additional harms of stigmatization, and the delivery of a poor quality of medical care obtained through the emergency room or from multiple providers [51]. This breakdown of trust between physician and patient may lead to a sense of desperation that leads patients to hoard medications or even purchase psychotropic drugs on the street [52]. Underlying the phenomena of pseudoaddiction are recent discoveries regarding the individual variation in pain sensitivity, metabolism of opioids, and the effect of gender, ethnicity, and cultural and temperamental differences in the experience and expression of pain [53–55]. Even when a patient has a true addiction and displays this behavior, it is not necessarily ethical to refuse controlled substances for established chronic pain. This is perhaps the most challenging of all the ethical dilemmas faced, and, from a clinical perspective, must be determined on a case-by-case basis.

Many patients who display some signs of addiction such as utilizing drugs for effects other than analgesia may have an undiagnosed depression or anxiety disorder. The Household Drug Survey found a high correlation between mental illness and substance abuse. Of adults with serious mental illness, 20.3% abused or were dependent upon alcohol or drugs, while the comparable statistic for persons without mental illness was 6.3%. During the last year 3.0 million adults were dually diagnosed [7]. A study of 37 patients with chronic pain found more than half of the patients had a history of one or more episodes of major depression and/or alcohol abuse before the onset of their chronic pain [56]. Treatment of the underlying mental or addictive illness may enable these patients to adhere to, and benefit from, even prolonged opioid therapy.

## Compassion, Autonomy, and Function in Patients with Chronic Pain

The core argument for providing patients with treatment for any condition revolves around the principles of beneficence and nonmaleficence, that is, trying to do good and trying not to do harm. These two principles form a hub around which other ethical principles and values such as autonomy, justice, respect for persons, confidentiality and informed consent rotate as spokes (fig. 1). Each of these principles will now be examined as they related to the treatment of chronic pain in persons with addictive disorders.

The principle of autonomy compels physicians to consider the patient's wishes, beliefs, and goals as part of medical decision making. Patients often wish to be relieved of distress when they are in pain even though the costs of utilizing opioids to obtain relief may be considerable such as deterioration in functioning which compromises quality of life. Patients developing SUD in the setting of chronic pain may often wish to compel their practitioners to provide medication even if the medication is causing harm including addiction. This introduces a major ethical dilemma into the care of patients with chronic pain.

Justice is another ethical issue that informs heath care decisions. This ethical principle compels us to provide care in a fair and just manner, and suggests that health care resources should not be distributed by physicians based on subjective factors such as race, ethnicity, lifestyle or economic resources, and that patients' social worth should not be used as a criterion to exclude them from legitimate clinical care, including pain treatment. Justice comes to the fore in three main areas of chronic pain treatment for patients with addictions: identification of patients with SUD as a separate and distinct class of persons, considering opioids as possessing biological and social characteristics that distinguish them from other medically useful pharmaceuticals, and isolating persons with addictions as different persons than those with other chronic diseases. Underlying each of these distinctions is the assumption that addiction is not a brain disease like other psychiatric illnesses [57]. Until very recently the general perception of addiction in government, law, and society was that it is a purely psychosocial and voluntary condition. Because of this significant inherent difference from other medical and even psychiatric conditions, addiction required differential treatment legally, politically, and socially. These differences influenced the attitudes and practices of segments of the medical profession resulting in unjust treatment of persons with addiction with and without chronic pain [58].

The latest statistics indicate that even if patients with chronic pain and SUD desire addiction treatment that might enable them to receive therapy for chronic pain, it may not be available. The cohort of persons with substance abuse or dependence that needed treatment, but were not able to receive it rose from 3.9 to 5.0 million in 2001. 377,000 people reported they felt the need for treatment and 101,000 of these had sought substance use treatment but were unable to obtain it [59]. The health care crises for the uninsured and working poor who are overrepresented in samples of both chronic pain and SUD patients compound the problem [60]. The physician's obligation to 'support access to health care for all people' is a principle of the AMA Code and is being given increasing attention in other statements of professional duties [61].

From a pharmacological perspective, differential prescribing laws may not be justified. It may be unjust to prevent addicted patients from gaining access to a physician prescription for methadone maintenance for addiction when the same physician can use it for another patient with chronic pain, and may be able to use it to treat both simultaneously. These contradictions reach their nadir in regulations pertaining to methadone. Currently only federally licensed narcotic treatment programs (MMTPs) can legally dispense methadone for purposes of maintenance or detoxification for opioid addiction. However, any physician with a valid Drug Enforcement Administration (DEA) license can prescribe methadone for chronic pain and this is considered a legitimate medical purpose.

These contradictory legal rulings and policy statements may leave clinicians feeling as if they are caught between the Scylla of having state medical boards investigate them for overprescribing and the Charybdis of being sued for undertreatment of pain [40]. Understanding the realities both legal and clinical of pain management and addiction, the use of judicious consultation and careful documentation of the rationale behind drug choice, taking precautions to manage drug misuse, and assuring continued benefit from therapy can assist physicians to avoid both extremes of treatment. There is also ample evidence that addiction is a stigmatizing condition negatively influencing the delivery of health care to patients with addiction. Link et al. [62] found a relatively strong and enduring effect of stigma on the well-being of patients with SUD and mental illness. Chronic pain and SUD are often coupled with other diseases like hepatitis C and HIV that are also stigmatizing [63].

These multiple sources of stigma create overlapping vulnerabilities, which warrant additional ethical safeguards in the treatment of chronic pain in the context of addiction [64]. Clinicians need to be sensitive to labeling patients as 'addicts' or 'substance abusers' and documenting such labels in the chart unless it will serve legitimate medical purposes such as facilitating proper treatment in the emergency room or arranging SUD therapy [65]. The use of urine toxicology and other addiction tools for assessment and monitoring are important aspects of comprehensive care for chronic pain patients with a history of addictions, but careful attention must be paid to educating patients about the purpose of these tools, and protecting their privacy [66, 67]. When patients do engage in the misuse or abuse of prescription narcotics, limits must be set and patients held accountable but this must be done in a way that continues to respect their humanity and self-determination.

This ethic of respect for persons has become one of the most challenging ethical issues in current medical practice. It directs us to respect patient autonomy and facilitate shared decision making which incorporates patient values, preferences, and goals. An aspect of respect for persons often neglected in the ethics of pain management is belief and trust in the credibility and integrity of the patient. Too often clinicians start an assessment of pain from a position of bias both personal and scientific [68]. It is well documented that medical training tends to see the objective and organic as 'real, true and significant' and the subjective and psychological as somehow 'unreal, false, and less important' [19, 69]. These terms have deep philosophical roots traced to the mind–body dualism of Greek philosophy and Descartes with their modern counterparts in clinician suspicion, disparagement, labeling, and rejection of patients with irritable bowel syndrome, fibromyalgia and other functional somatic syndromes [69–71]. Edwards [20] has said that when clinicians fail to respect the person of the pain patient, 'Medical professionalism then become inflictors of pain rather than pain relievers'. Contemporary research in psychosomatic medicine, much of it conducted in consultation-liaison psychiatry, has questioned these distinctions and supported an integrative approach to pain assessment and management that utilizes the best of modern diagnostic technology while honoring the validity and truthfulness of the patient's experience [72, 73].

A corollary of respect for persons is honoring and protecting the privacy and confidentiality of patient's medical information. Physicians need to be aware of the special regulations and protections for substance abuse information, particularly in the light of the new Health Insurance Portability and Accountability Act (HIPAA) mandates [74]. They need also to realize the enormous potential negative consequences of documenting addiction or even a positive toxicology for employment, education, security clearance, health and life insurance, as well as family relationships. An essential but often overlooked part of chronic pain treatment for persons with addiction is being clear at the onset of care about the limitations and protections for confidentiality. Patients who are receiving treatment under the auspices of third-party payers, the criminal justice system, or as part of occupational health must be educated about the dual roles of the providers involved and the restrictions on confidentiality [67, 75]. Clinicians may be faced with difficult decisions such as whether to report drug diversion or prescription forgery to the authorities. Family members may be allies in the patient's treatment and yet physicians cannot speak to them without the patient's explicit permission except in emergency situations. They must be careful to protect both the family member and the patient if they choose to act on the information. Suicidal and homicidal impulses, child abuse, domestic violence, and driving under the influence are not uncommon in chronic pain and SUD and physicians must inform themselves and patients of the legal and ethical mandates allowing breaches of confidentiality and privacy in such cases [76, 77].

The ethic of autonomy and respect for persons are operationalized in the doctrine of informed consent. Informed consent encompasses the capacity to understand the risks, benefits, and alternatives of a treatment, to communicate a choice regarding therapy, to deliberate and reason about the consequences of the proposed medication, and to appreciate how the treatment will affect life and values. Finally decisions must be made in the absence of strong internal or external coercion [78]. Informed consent is the premise behind the widely used opioid contract which is a valuable aid in maintaining patients with a history or current problem with chemical dependency in chronic pain treatment [79]. The degree to which addiction is voluntary is a very old debate recently revived. Evidence from basic science studies of the pathophysiology and pharmacology of both chronic pain and addiction, and from neuroimaging and molecular genetics suggests that both the cognitive and volitional capacities required for informed consent are diminished in patients with addiction and chronic pain to varying degrees [57]. The behavioral phenomena that characterize SUD, compulsion, obsession, loss of control, craving, and the continuation of substance use despite negative, medical, psychological, and social consequences are understood from this perspective as symptoms of a brain disease [57, 80]. The neuropsychiatric correlates of these behaviors, neuroadaptation and sensitization, appear to diminish the authentic freedom and decisional capacity of the addicted individual as they pertain to informed consent [81]. It is widely recognized that stress, sleep deprivation, anxiety, trauma, and depression or other psychological factors that often accompany pain and SUD may both lower the pain threshold and diminish decisional capacity and autonomy [1, 82].

The practical implication of these theoretical findings is that patients with a history of substance abuse or an active problem may enter into opioid contracts with good intentions but diminished capacity for informed consent. If aware of these limitations in the patient's voluntarism, physicians can provide additional safeguards to protect the patient against relapse or development of addiction such as involving partners and family in treatment, dispensing only small amounts of medication, early and consistent collaboration with substance abuse experts, and most importantly establishing an open and trusting relationship in which patients feel safe expressing cravings, lapses, and temptations [83]. Regarding minor infractions of the opioid contract as slips expected in a chronic and relapsing disease rather than intentional undermining of treatment allows both physician and patient to arrive at more constructive solutions. Physicians must also be vigilant about diagnosing and treating the common psychiatric conditions associated with chronic pain that can further reduce decisional capacity such as depression, anxiety and psychosis [18].

## A Harm Reduction Approach

Physicians involved in the care of patients with active or historical SUD and chronic pain are confronted with a number of ethical dilemmas. The following recommendations constitute a harm reduction approach to the care of patients with addiction and chronic pain [84]. Harm reduction is a philosophy and a practice utilized in some segments of the addiction medicine community [85]. It offers a means of managing many of the dilemmas patients with chronic pain and addiction present [86, 87].

Portenoy [2] and Miotto et al. [88] have identified a variety of factors that signal problematic SUD use in the chronic pain environment (table 4). None of these have been subjected to controlled clinical trials and can substitute for the casuistry of the independent clinical judgment. Notwithstanding their limitations, failure to explore, document and address these risk factors would not meet the standard of care for treating chronic pain patients with addiction [88, 89].

***Table 4.*** Warning signs [adapted from 88]

Mild misuse
    Increasing dose without permission occasionally[1]
    Occasional loss of prescription
    Preference for a specific pain formulation
Moderate misuse
    Use of the drug to treat symptoms other than chronic pain[2]
    Use of alcohol or other illicit drugs[2]
    Stockpiling drug[1]
    Occasional request for early refill without purported loss of medication[1]
    Purchasing drugs on the street once or twice[1,2]
    Seeking prescriptions from other providers or the emergency room infrequently but
      informing primary clinician[1]
    Complaints of adverse effects with any but preferred pain medication
    Seeking the psychoactive rather than analgesic effects of medication[2]
    Nonadherence to psychosocial dimensions of pain program
    Inordinate amount of time and energy spent in assuring adequate supply and dosage of
      pain medication[1]
    Decline in functioning from pretreatment baseline
Severe misuses
    Injecting oral formulations
    Stealing drugs
    Forging prescriptions
    Continual escalation of dosage
    Diversion of medications
    Consistent pattern of purchasing drugs on the street
    Seeking prescriptions from other providers or the emergency room frequently
    Either hiding behavior or lying to primary clinician about sources and frequency of
      obtaining medications from other sources
    Refusal to participate in any psychosocial aspects of pain program
    Refusing addiction treatment
    Dysfunctional behavior or gross decline in functioning in multiple spheres of life

[1] Behaviors that may also be associated with pseudoaddiction.
[2] Behaviors that may also be associated with inadequately treated psychiatric disorders.

Researchers disagree on the classification, significance and gravity of the various factors, particularly those on the less pathological end of the spectrum. Table 3 lists some of the most common factors according to whether they represent mild, moderate or severe misuse of controlled substances [89]. Mild misuse is an occasional patient-initiated adjustment in prescribed regimen; moderate misuse is a more frequent and severe misuse of prescriptions contrary to the physician's intentions and instructions; pathological use involves exploitation of the physician and often criminal behavior. The frequency, contextual features, intentionality of the patient, and severity of the factors must all be considered when formulating an appropriate therapeutic response to problematic behavior [88].

In every situation in which a problematic behavior emerges such as escalating the dose of medication without permission, consider how best to use the behavior therapeutically. Explore with the patient their rationale and objectives for the action. Were they afraid that if they told the physician they were in pain, he would think they were addicted and further reduce or stop the medication altogether or were they seeking additional relief from anxiety? In the first case reassurance should be the response and a readjustment of dose, in the second the patient may require assessment and treatment of an anxiety disorder as well a substance abuse. Patients with drug misuse or even abuse may respond to an increase in visits, closer monitoring with urine drug screens, pain diary, psychiatric assessment, tighter control of medication supplies or other strategies [90]. Pseudoaddictive behaviors or those associated with other mental illnesses will usually respond to the appropriate pharmacological and psychosocial therapy, while true addiction will continue to escalate and declare itself with an ever more exploitative and dangerous pattern. Even when a patient's behavior necessitates curtailment of narcotics for the protection of patient and community, providers must not abandon patients but continue to offer health maintenance and prevention and therapy for the many medical consequences of substance use.

## Steps for the Ethical Management of Pain

The following recommendations based on the work of experts in pain medicine offer a harm reduction approach to the ethical issues examined [18, 40]. (1) The cornerstone of management is to establish the pathophysiology of the pain where possible and the appropriate indications for pain treatment. (2) Reasonable trials of nonpharmacological treatments and nonopioid analgesia are recommended. (3) If controlled substances are considered necessary, addiction is less likely with long-acting formulations such as sustained release morphine than short-acting drugs like oxycodone, and prescription of round-the-clock pain relief rather than as-needed also reduces the reinforcement which comes from medications. (4) Tolerance is unusual with opioids and generally reflects changes in underlying pathophysiology or metabolism warranting investigation. (5) Patients with a history of SUD or active use may require higher doses of pain relief. (6) There are documented individual variations in the types and dosages of pain medications required for analgesia. (7) Teach patients that there is no absolute cure for addiction or chronic pain, that both are life-long struggles with relapses and recoveries. (8) Help patients to develop

---

realistic expectations about the benefits and side effects of medications that will temper their inclinations to alter the regimen, or seek psychoactive alternatives either licitly or illicitly. (9) Utilize pain ratings and physical performance but supplement these with overall quality of life and functioning measures. (10) Employ other modalities such as physical therapy, self-help groups like AA and Narcotics Anonymous (NA), and family therapy to obtain a more holistic and balanced treatment plan.

## Conclusion

While seeking to provide empirically based chronic pain regimens clinicians must be cognizant and responsive to legal mandates and professional standards which may at times conflict with the higher ethical duty to provide compassionate and humane care for persons with dual diagnoses. Sensitivity and training in identifying and addressing the clinical instantiation of the cardinal ethical principles and values of beneficence, nonmaleficence, autonomy, justice, respect for persons, confidentiality, and informed consent can enable physicians to offer care that is well-grounded in the contemporary science and sound ethical analysis. A harm reduction approach to the treatment of patients with chronic pain in the context of addiction does not guarantee a successful outcome but may contribute to the minimization of harm and the maximization of benefit for this often inadequately treated group of patients.

## Acknowledgments

The author wishes to thank Christina Martinez, MD, Joan Gibson, PhD and Michael Bogenschutz, MD for reviewing drafts of this chapter.

## References

1   Savage SR: Addiction in the treatment of pain: Significance, recognition, and management. J Pain Symptom Manage 1993;8/5:265–278.
2   Portenoy RK: Chronic opioid therapy in nonmalignant pain. J Pain Symptom Manage 1990; 5(1 suppl):S46–S62.
3   Gilson AM, Joranson DE: U.S. policies relevant to the prescribing of opioid analgesics for the treatment of pain in patients with addictive disease. Clin J Pain 2002;18(4 suppl):S91–S98.
4   Portenoy RK, Dole V, Joseph H, Lowinson J, Rice C, Segal S, Richman BL: Pain management and chemical dependency. Evolving perspectives. JAMA 1997;278:592–593.
5   Wise MG, Rundell JR: Textbook of Consultation-Liaison Psychiatry. Washington, American Psychiatric Publishing, 2002.
6   Leeman CP: Psychiatric consultations and ethics consultations. Similarities and differences. Gen Hosp Psychiatry 2000;22/4:270–275.

7    Substance Abuse and Mental Health Services Administration: 2001 National Household Survey on Drug Abuse, 2001. http://www.samhsa.gov/oas/nhsda.htm

8    Rice DP: Economic costs of substance abuse, 1995. Proc Assoc Am Physicians 1999;111/2: 119–125.

9    Weaver M, Schnoll S: Abuse liability in opioid therapy for pain treatment in patients with an addiction history. Clin J Pain 2002;18(4 suppl):S61–S69.

10   Fishbain DA, Rosomoff HL, Rosomoff RS: Drug abuse, dependence, and addiction in chronic pain patients. Clin J Pain 1992;8/2:77–85.

11   Rosenblum A, Joseph H, Fong C, Kipnis S, Cleland C, Portenoy RK: Prevalence and characteristics of chronic pain among chemically dependent patients in methadone maintenance and residential treatment facilities. JAMA 2003;289:2370–2378.

12   American Academy of Pain Medicine and American Pain Society Consensus Statement: The use of opioids for the treatment of chronic pain. Clin J Pain 1997;13:6–8.

13   Joranson DE: Federal and state regulation of opioids. J Pain Symptom Manage 1990;5(1 suppl): S12–S23.

14   Hicks RD: Pain management in the chemically dependent patient. Hawaii Med J 1989;48: 491–492, 494–495.

15   Sulmasy DP, Haller K, Terry PB: More talk, less paper: Predicting the accuracy of substituted judgments. Am J Med 1994;96:432–438.

16   Sugarman J, McCrory DC, Powell D, Krasny A, Adams B, Ball E, Cassell C: Empirical research on informed consent. An annotated bibliography. Hastings Cent Rep 1999;29/1:S1–S42.

17   Cohen MJ, Jasser S, Herron PD, Margolis CG: Ethical perspectives: Opioid treatment of chronic pain in the context of addiction. Clin J Pain 2002;18(4 suppl):S99–S107.

18   Pappagallo M, Heinberg LJ: Ethical issues in the management of chronic nonmalignant pain. Semin Neurol 1997;17/3:203–211.

19   Dugan DC: Pain and the ethics of pain management. HEC Forum 1996;8:330–339.

20   Edwards RB: Pain and the ethics of pain management. Soc Sci Med 1984;18:515–523

21   Rich BA: A legacy of silence: Bioethics and the culture of pain. J Med Humanit 1997;18/4:233–259.

22   Kirsh KL, Whitcomb LA, Donaghy K, Passik SD: Abuse and addiction issues in medically ill patients with pain: Attempts at clarification of terms and empirical study. Clin J Pain 2002; 18(4 suppl):S52–S60.

23   American Academy of Pain Medicine, American Pain Society, Medicine, American Society of Addiction Medicine: Definitions Related to the Use of Opioids for the Treatment of Pain, 2001. http://www.asam.org/ppol/paindef.htm

24   Beauchamp TL, Childress JF: Principles of Biomedical Ethics. New York, Oxford University Press, 2001.

25   Lloyd GER: Hippocratic Writings. London, Penguin Books, 1983.

26   Jonsen AR, Seigler M, Winslade WJ: Clinical Ethics. New York, McGraw-Hill, 1998.

27   The use of opioids for the treatment of chronic pain. A consensus statement from the American Academy of Pain Medicine and the American Pain Society. Clin J Pain 1997;13/1:6–8.

28   Passik SD, Weinreb HJ: Managing chronic nonmalignant pain: Overcoming obstacles to the use of opioids. Adv Ther 2000;17/2:70–83.

29   Chabal C, Erjavec MK, Jacobson L, Mariano A, Chaney E: Prescription opiate abuse in chronic pain patients: Clinical criteria, incidence, and predictors. Clin J Pain 1997;13/2:150–155.

30   Bailey DN: Drug use in patients admitted to a university trauma center: Results of limited (rather than comprehensive) toxicology screening. J Anal Toxicol 1990;14/1:22–24.

31   National Institute on Alcohol and Alcoholism: Eighth Special Report to the U.S. Congress on Alcohol and Health, 1993.

32   Kennedy JA, Crowley TJ: Chronic pain and substance abuse: A pilot study of opioid maintenance. J Subst Abuse Treat 1990;7/4:233–238.

33   Currie SR, Hodgins DC, Crabtree A, Jacobi J, Armstrong S: Outcome from integrated pain management treatment for recovering substance abusers. J Pain 2003;4/2:91–100.

34   Dunbar SA, Katz NP: Chronic opioid therapy for nonmalignant pain in patients with a history of substance abuse: Report of 20 cases. J Pain Symptom Manage 1996;11/3:163–171.

35  Pisano DJ: Controlled substances and pain management: Regulatory oversight, formularies, and cost decisions. J Law Med Ethics 1996;24:310–316.

36  Bendtsen P, Hensing G, Ebeling C, Schedin A: What are the qualities of dilemmas experienced when prescribing opioids in general practice? Pain 1999;82/1:89–96.

37  Rupp H, Maisch B, Brilla CG: Drug withdrawal and rebound hypertension: Differential action of the central antihypertensive drugs moxonidine and clonidine. Cardiovasc Drugs Ther 1996;10(suppl 1):251–262.

38  Albert T: Suit targets Paxil ads, tests FDA authority. AMNews, September 2002.

39  Zajecka J, Tracy KA, Mitchell S: Discontinuation symptoms after treatment with serotonin reuptake inhibitors: A literature review. J Clin Psychiatry 1997;58/7:291–297.

40  Savage SR: Opioid therapy of chronic pain: Assessment of consequences. Acta Anaesthesiol Scand 1999;43:909–917.

41  Nemeroff CB: The rational use of narcotic analgesics, benzodiazepines and psychostimulants in medical practice. A response to the paper 'Prescribing Addictive Medication'. N C Med J 1990;51/5:240–243.

42  Katz N, Fanciullo GJ: Role of urine toxicology testing in the management of chronic opioid therapy. Clin J Pain 2002;18(4 suppl):S76–S82.

43  Sees KL, Clark HW: Opioid use in the treatment of chronic pain: Assessment of addiction. J Pain Symptom Manage 1993;8/5:257–264.

44  Breitbart W, Rosenfeld BD, Passik SD, McDonald MV, Thaler H, Portenoy RK: The undertreatment of pain in ambulatory AIDS patients. Pain 1996;65/2–3:243–249.

45  Albert T: Doctor guilty of elder abuse for undertreating pain. AMNews, July 2001.

46  Council on Ethical and Judicial Affairs: Code of Medical Ethics. Chicago, American Medical Association, 2002.

47  Vaillant GE: The beginning of wisdom is never calling a patient a borderline; or the clinical management of immature defenses in the treatment of individuals with personality disorders. J Psychother Pract Res 1992;1:117–134.

48  Groves JE: Taking care of the hateful patient. N Engl J Med 1978;298:883–887.

49  Jackson JL, Kroenke K: Difficult patient encounters in the ambulatory clinic: Clinical predictors and outcomes. Arch Intern Med 1999;159:1069–1075.

50  Weissman DE, Haddox JD: Opioid pseudoaddiction – An iatrogenic syndrome. Pain 1989;36:363–366.

51  Hung CI, Liu CY, Chen CY, Yang CH, Yeh EK: Meperidine addiction or treatment frustration? Gen Hosp Psychiatry 2001;23/1:31–35.

52  Weissman DE: Understanding pseudoaddiction. J Pain Symptom Manage 1994;9/2:74.

53  Elmer GI, Pieper JO, Negus SS, Woods JH: Genetic variance in nociception and its relationship to the potency of morphine-induced analgesia in thermal and chemical tests. Pain 1998;75/1:129–140.

54  Fillingim RB, Doleys DM, Edwards RR, Lowery D: Clinical characteristics of chronic back pain as a function of gender and oral opioid use. Spine 2003;28/2:143–150.

55  Bates MS, Edwards WT, Anderson KO: Ethnocultural influences on variation in chronic pain perception. Pain 1993;52/1:101–112.

56  Katon W, Egan K, Miller D: Chronic pain: Lifetime psychiatric diagnoses and family history. Am J Psychiatry 1985;142:1156–1160.

57  Wise RA: Addiction becomes a brain disease. Neuron 2000;26/1:27–33.

58  Turk DC, Brody MC, Okifuji EA: Physicians' attitudes and practices regarding the long-term prescribing of opioids for non-cancer pain. Pain 1994;59/2:201–208.

59  Drake RE, Essock SM, Shaner A, Carey KB, Minkoff K, Kola L, Lynde D, Osher FC, Clark RE, Rickards L: Implementing dual diagnosis services for clients with severe mental illness. Psychiatr Serv 2001;52:469–476.

60  McManus SM, Pohl CM: Ethics and financing: Overview of the U.S. health care system. J Health Hum Resour Adm 1994;16:332–349.

61  ABIM Foundation. American Board of Internal Medicine; ACP-ASIM Foundation. American College of Physicians-American Society of Internal Medicine; European Federation of Internal

Medicine: Medical professionalism in the new millennium: A physician charter. Ann Intern Med 2002;136/3:243–246.

62  Link BG, Struening EL, Rahav M, Phelan JC, Nuttbrock L: On stigma and its consequences: Evidence from a longitudinal study of men with dual diagnoses of mental illness and substance abuse. J Health Soc Behav 1997;38/2:177–190.

63  HIV-related knowledge and stigma – United States, 2000. MMWR Morb Mortal Wkly Rep 2000; 49:1062–1064.

64  McGovern TF: Vulnerability: Reflection on its ethical implications for the protection of participants in SAMHSA programs. Ethics Behav 1998;8:293–304.

65  Cunningham JA, Sobell LC, Chow VM: What's in a label? The effects of substance types and labels on treatment considerations and stigma. J Stud Alcohol 1993;54:693–699.

66  Giannini AJ, Giannini JN: Historical, ethical, and legal issues in mandatory drug testing. JONAS Healthc Law Ethics Regul 2000;2/4:105–107, 111.

67  Forrest AR: Ethical aspects of workplace urine screening for drug abuse. J Med Ethics 1997;23/1: 12–17.

68  Bates MS, Rankin-Hill L, Sanchez-Ayendez M: The effects of the cultural context of health care on treatment of and response to chronic pain and illness. Soc Sci Med 1997;45:1433–1447.

69  Gordon LE: Mental health of medical students: The culture of objectivity in medicine. Pharos 1996;59/2:2–10.

70  Hazemeijer I, Rasker JJ: Fibromyalgia and the therapeutic domain. A philosophical study on the origins of fibromyalgia in a specific social setting. Rheumatology (Oxford) 2003;42:507–515.

71  Kirsner JB: The irritable bowel syndrome. A clinical review and ethical considerations. Arch Intern Med 1981;141:635–639.

72  Turk DC, Okifuji A: Assessment of patients' reporting of pain: An integrated perspective. Lancet 1999;353:1784–1788.

73  Kornfeld DS: Consultation-liaison psychiatry: Contributions to medical practice. Am J Psychiatry 2002;159:1964–1972.

74  Felthous AR: Substance abuse and the duty to protect. Bull Am Acad Psychiatry Law 1993;21: 419–426.

75  Tilton SH: Right to privacy and confidentiality of medical records. Occup Med 1996;11/1:17–29.

76  McCrady BS, Bux DA Jr: Ethical issues in informed consent with substance abusers. J Consult Clin Psychol 1999;67:186–193.

77  Leeman CP, Cohen MA, Parkas V: Should a psychiatrist report a bus driver's alcohol and drug abuse? An ethical dilemma. Gen Hosp Psychiatry 2001;23:333–336.

78  Roberts LW: Informed Consent and Psychiatric Care; in Smelser NJ, Baltes PB (eds): International Encyclopedia of the Social and Behavioral Sciences. Amsterdam, Elsevier Science, 2001.

79  Roberts LW, Warner TD, Brody JL, Roberts B, Lauriello J, Lyketsos C: Patient and psychiatrist ratings of hypothetical schizophrenia research protocols: Assessment of harm potential and factors influencing participation decisions. Am J Psychiatry 2002;159:573–584.

80  Robinson TE, Berridge KC: The psychology and neurobiology of addiction: An incentive-sensitization view. Addiction 2000;95(suppl 2):S91–S117.

81  Roberts LW: Addiction and consent. Am J Bioeth 2002;2/2:58–60.

82  Kuch K: Psychological factors and the development of chronic pain. Clin J Pain 2001;17(4 suppl): S33–S38.

83  Roberts LW: Informed consent and the capacity for voluntarism. Am J Psychiatry 2002;159: 705–712.

84  Carey KB, Purnine DM, Maisto SA, Carey MP, Simons JS: Treating substance abuse in the context of severe and persistent mental illness: Clinicians' perspectives. J Subst Abuse Treat 2000;19/2:189–198.

85  Marlatt GA: Harm reduction: Come as you are. Addict Behav 1996;21:779–788.

86  Hamilton M: Researching harm reduction – Care and contradictions. Subst Use Misuse 1999; 34/1:119–141.

87  Hathaway AD: Shortcomings of harm reduction: Toward a morally invested drug reform strategy. Int J Drug Policy 2001;12/2:125–137.

88 Miotto K, Compton P, Ling W, Conolly M: Diagnosing addictive disease in chronic pain patients. Psychosomatics 1996;37/3:223–235.

89 Longo LP, Parran T Jr, Johnson B, Kinsey W: Addiction. II. Identification and management of the drug-seeking patient. Am Fam Physician 2000;61:2401–2408.

90 Nedeljkovic SS, Wasan A, Jamison RN: Assessment of efficacy of long-term opioid therapy in pain patients with substance abuse potential. Clin J Pain 2002;18(4 suppl):S39–S51.

Cynthia M.A. Geppert, MD, PhD
Attending Psychiatrist, New Mexico Veterans Affairs Health Care System,
Assistant Professor, Department of Psychiatry, University of New Mexico,
New Mexico Veterans Affairs Health Care System
1501 San Pedro Dr. SE, Albuquerque, NM 87108 (USA)
Tel. +1 505 265 1711, ext. 5551, Fax +1 505 256 5443, E-Mail doc@ethicdoc.com

# Subject Index

Activities of daily living (ADLs)
    prospects, disability studies 57, 58
    rheumatoid arthritis, impact 44, 45
Addiction
    assessment 129
    availability of chronic pain treatment
      161, 162
    definition 129, 157
    monitoring, opioid users 129–131
    opioids 128–131
    prevalence, chronic pain population 129
    pseudoaddiction behaviors 159, 160
A$\delta$-fibers, nociception 80
Alcohol abuse, *see also* Substance abuse
    chronic pain patients 155
    pain relief, impact 156
Amygdala, nociception 84
Anger reduction, alleviation of pain 35, 36
Antidepressants, pain management 67
Anxiety
    complex regional pain syndrome
      comorbidity 93
    reduction/alleviation of pain 34, 35
Autonomy, chronic pain treatment 160,
    161, 163

Basal ganglia, nociception 84
Battle fatigue, *see* Gulf War syndrome;
    Postwar syndromes
Behaviors, pain and depression treatment
    considerations 15–19
Beneficence, definition 155, 157

Calcium channel blockers, opioid
    combination therapy 127
Catastrophizing, effects on pain and
    depression 14, 16, 66
Causalgia, *see* Complex regional pain
    syndrome
Cerebellum, nociception 84
C-fibers, nociception 80, 81
Classical conditioning, pain 30
Clonidine, opioid combination therapy
    128
Cognition
    opioid side effects 132, 133
    psychological behaviorism theory, pain
      30, 31
Cognitive behavioral theory (CBT)
    chronic pain treatment 11, 12, 65
    components 11
Complex regional pain syndrome (CRPS)
    caregiver strain and stress 94
    central nervous system dysfunction 98,
      99
    diagnosis 91
    disability levels 94
    etiopathogenesis 91, 92
    motor dysfunction 98
    nomenclature 90, 91
    psychiatric comorbidity
      anxiety 93
      depression 93
      factitious disorder 94
      neglect 94, 95

overview 92, 93
  substance abuse 93
quality of life 96
sensory disturbances 98
stressful life events 96
sympathetic nervous system dysfunction 96–98
treatment algorithm 99
types 89
validity, reflex sympathetic dystrophy 90
Coping
  definition 14
  effects on depression and pain 66
  effects on disability levels 14

Depression
  chronic pain comorbidity 3, 7, 131, 132
  complex regional pain syndrome
    comorbidity 93
  definition 1
  demoralization comparison 9
  disability prediction, pain 8
  etiology 5–7
  incidence, medical diseases 7
  treatment, suffering perspectives
    behaviors 15–19
    dimensions 12–15
    diseases 6–9
    life stories 9–12
    overview 4, 5
Diathesis-stress model, pain-depression
  interactions 12, 13
Dimensional perspective, pain and
  depression treatment considerations
  12–15
Disability
  complex regional pain syndrome levels 94
  function-psychological well-being
    linkage 47–49, 51–53
  intervention points, rheumatoid arthritis
    54–57
  life activity grouping, assessment 44
  models 42–44
  personal value concept, disability
    assessment 45–47
  postwar syndrome prevention 112, 113
  prospects for study 57, 58

Dorsal horn, pain neurobiology 81–83
Drug Enforcement Administration (DEA),
  considerations in opioid prescription
  142, 143

Emotion, psychological behaviorism theory
  of pain 33

Factitious disorder, complex regional pain
  syndrome comorbidity 94
Fear-avoidance beliefs, pain outcome
  effects 16, 17

Genetics, pain depression linkage 69,
  70–72
Glutamate, nociceptive processing 83
Gulf War syndrome, *see also* Postwar
  syndromes
  epidemiological studies 103
  incidence 103
  symptoms 103, 105

Hypothalamus, nociception 84

Internalizing-externalizing (IE) structural
  model
  comorbidity, psychopathological
    syndromes 64, 65
  pain relevance 72–74

Joint Commission on Accreditation of
  Healthcare Organizations (JCAHO),
  considerations in opioid prescription
  143
Justice
  chronic pain treatment 160, 161
  definition, substance abuse 157

Learning, psychological behaviorism
  theory of pain 30
Life stories, pain and depression treatment
  considerations 9–12

N-methyl-*D*-aspartate (NMDA)
  antagonists, opioid combination therapy
    126, 127, 133
  pain neurobiology 82, 83, 127

Minnesota Multiphasic Personality Inventory (MMPI), chronic pain effects 13

Neglect, complex regional pain syndrome comorbidity 94, 95
Neurokinin
    knockout mouse studies, pain and emotion 71, 72
    pain neurotransmission 80
    receptor 71
Nimodipine, opioid combination therapy 127
Nociceptin, knockout mouse studies, pain and emotion 72
Nonmaleficence, definition 155, 157
Norepinephrine, pain and depression modulation 68

Opioids
    addiction 128–131
    behavioral influences 159
    cancer pain management 124
    cognitive side effects 132, 133
    efficacy factors, chronic pain management
        analgesia versus side effects 124
        controversies, efficacy 144, 145
        drug-centered characteristics 126–128
        pain-centered characteristics 125, 126
        patient-centered characteristics 125
    ethics, pain management 153, 154
    low-dose antagonists, potency enhancement 128
    primary care physician management of chronic pain
        criminal justice system considerations 142, 158, 159
        Drug Enforcement Administration considerations 142, 143
        guideline inadequacy 144, 147
        Joint Commission on Accreditation of Healthcare Organizations guidelines 143
        medical board requirements 143
        patient-related issues 139–141
        pharmaceutical company marketing 143, 144

physician-related issues 141, 142
        pressures for/against prescribing 139
        resource availability and education 145–147
        risks, history of substance abuse 156–159
    substance abuse pain patient management, *see* Substance abuse
    tolerance 129, 130

Pain
    classification 2
    definitions 1, 2, 29
    depression comorbidity 3, 7
    neurobiology
        ascending tract and descending inhibition mechanisms 84, 85
        dorsal horn mechanisms 81–83
        overview 78, 79
        peripheral mechanisms 80, 81
    prevalence, chronic pain comorbidity 2, 123, 131, 132
    psychiatric disorder comorbidity 3
    treatment
        goals 3, 4
        suffering perspectives
            behaviors 15–19
            dimensions 12–15
            diseases 6–9
            life stories 9–12
            overview 4, 5
Pain behavior, psychological behaviorism theory of pain 32
Parietal lobe, nociception 84
Personality, psychological behaviorism theory of pain 31, 32
Physical dependence, definition 157
Physical therapy, pain outcome effects 17
Postwar syndromes, *see also* Gulf War syndrome
    disability prevention 112, 113
    epidemiological studies 103, 104
    health information systems 114, 115
    intensive rehabilitative care 113, 114
    population-based care 106–108

preclinical prevention 108–110
predisposing, precipitating, and
    perpetuating factors 105
prevention strategy implementation by
    Department of Defense
    health services research agenda
        and expertise development 116,
        117
    'Operation Solace' following
        September 11 Pentagon attack 118,
        119
    primary care practice guidelines on
        postdeployment healthcare delivery
        117, 118
primary care mitigation of symptoms
    110–113
Preproenkephalin, knockout mouse studies,
    pain and emotion 72
Pseudoaddiction, behaviors 159, 160
Psychological behaviorism theory of pain
    overview 28, 29
    realms of pain investigation
        biology 29, 30
        cognition 30, 31
        emotion 33
        learning 30
        pain behavior 32
        personality 31, 32
        social environment 32, 33
    supporting research
        anger reduction and alleviation of pain
            35, 36
        anxiety reduction and alleviation of
            pain 34, 35
        psychological behaviorism therapy
            treatment of osteoarthritic pain 36,
            37
        sexual fantasy alleviation of pain 33,
            34
Psychological behaviorism theory of
    placebo
    overview 37
    pain studies
        pain anxiety and responsiveness 38,
            39
        pain sensitivity response 38
        study groups 37, 38

Psychological behaviorism therapy (PBT),
    treatment of osteoarthritic pain 36, 37

Reflex sympathetic dystrophy, *see* Complex
    regional pain syndrome
Rheumatoid arthritis (RA)
    disability models 42–44
    functional limitation assessment 44,
        45
    function-psychological well-being
        linkage 47–49, 51–53
    intervention points, disability 54–57
    personal value concept, disability
        assessment 45–47

Self-efficacy beliefs
    effects on depression and pain 66
    pain outcome effects 15, 16
Sensitization, pain neurobiology 82
Serotonin, pain and depressoin modulation
    68
Sexual fantasy, alleviation of pain 33,
    34
Shell shock, *see* Gulf War syndrome;
    Postwar syndromes
Social environment, psychological
    behaviorism theory of pain 32, 33
Somatosensory cortex, nociception 84
Substance abuse, *see also* Addiction;
    Alcohol abuse; Opioids
    complex regional pain syndrome
        comorbidity 93
    diagnostic criteria 18
    excessive self-administration of
        medications 18
    opioid prescription considerations,
        chronic pain management
        autonomy 160, 161, 163
        availability of pain treatment 161,
            162
        core ethical conflict 154–160
        harm reduction approach 164–166
        justice 160, 161
        overview 139, 140, 151, 152
        privacy and confidentiality 163
        psychological comorbidity 163,
            164

Substance abuse (continued)
    steps in ethical management of pain
        166, 167
    warning signs of abuse 164, 165
    pain relief impact 156
    prevalence
        chronic pain population 18, 19, 129,
            152, 153
        United States 152
    risks, chronic pain treatment 156–158
Substance P
    antagonists, pain management 67, 68
    depression, role 70
    pain neurotransmission 80, 81
Suicide, chronic pain risks 8

Tachykinin, depression role 70
Tolerance
    definition 157
    opioids 129, 130

Valued life activities (VDLs)
    definition 41
    function-psychological well-being
        linkage 47–49, 51–53
    intervention points, rheumatoid arthritis
        54–57
    personal value concept, disability
        assessment 45–47
    prospects, disability studies 57, 58
    rheumatoid arthritis, impact 44, 45